THE ROCK CARLING FELLOWSHIP

1985

A difficult balance

EDITORIAL PEER REVIEW
IN MEDICINE

THE ROCK CARLING FELLOWSHIP

1985

A DIFFICULT BALANCE

EDITORIAL PEER REVIEW IN MEDICINE

Stephen Lock
MA, MSC, MB, FRCP
Editor, *British Medical Journal*

THE NUFFIELD
PROVINCIAL HOSPITALS TRUST
1985

Published by the
Nuffield Provincial Hospitals Trust
3 Prince Albert Road, London NW1 7SP

ISBN 0 900574 56 9

©Nuffield Provincial Hospitals Trust, 1985

Designed by Bernard Crossland
PRINTED IN GREAT BRITAIN BY
BURGESS & SON (ABINGDON) LTD
ABINGDON OXFORDSHIRE

CONTENTS

Contents

LIST OF FIGURES
AND TABLES

FIGURES

TABLES

List of figures and tables

And in that same hour, as they feasted
      Came forth fingers of a man's hand
          And the King saw
The part of the hand that wrote

And this was the writing that was written:
Mene, mene, tekel, upharsin
'Thou art weighed in the balance and found
  wanting.'

Text selected from the Bible
by Osbert Sitwell for *Belshazzar's Feast*
by William Walton

PREFACE

In the early 1890s the distinguished physicist Lord Rayleigh was leafing through some writings of J. J. Waterston, an unknown worker, and came across references to an unpublished paper in the archives of the Royal Society (1). Rayleigh obtained the manuscript, which had been submitted in 1845, and realized that Waterston should have had the priority subsequently given to Joule, Clausius, and Clark Maxwell. The work had been sent for peer review (the assessment of work by outside experts). One of the referees had been among the best qualified of the day, yet he had reported that 'the paper is nothing but nonsense, unfit even for reading before the Society'. Another had stated: 'the original principle itself involves an assumption which seems to me very difficult to admit, and by no means a satisfactory basis for a mathematical theory. . . .'

This anecdote might suggest that peer review is ineffective, at least for recognizing strikingly new work. Without more evidence such a generalization is not justified, but this episode is a reminder of how little one of the most important features of the editorial process has been studied.

Since its beginning peer review has had many proponents and critics, with a host of anecdotal accounts and theoretical suggestions. Nevertheless, few rigorous studies have been done, and Ingelfinger's statement of 20 years ago remains true: 'that data on the performance of the reviewing system are lacking is all the more astounding in view of the momentous influence the system exerts on the lives of those who write biomedical articles.' (2).

For this reason I welcomed the invitation by the Rock Carling trustees to discuss the issue. The Nuffield Provincial Hospitals Trust has a long tradition of emphasizing the value of audit of both process and outcome, and peer review is one of the key processes at several stages of scientific

References begin on p. 152

research—applications for a research grant, assessing an abstract of a contribution submitted to a meeting of a scientific society, and refereeing a paper for publication in a journal. Without publication, which entails such preliminary validation (continued afterwards by the journal's general and specialist readers), science cannot advance. And ensuring that peer review is as accurate, fair, and quick as possible in one of the principal tasks of most scientific editors (though they have other important roles, such as ensuring a balance in their journals between subjects, original *v* review articles, topical *v* archival contributions, and allocating the limited amount of space available).

Customarily here a Rock Carling lecturer should thank his sponsors and give his credentials. The first task is easier than the second. From their inception I have admired the Rock Carling lectures, not only for the choice of speaker and subject but also for the elegance with which the latter has been handled and the subsequent translations of the principles proposed into action. Thus I am particularly grateful to the trust for asking me to give this lecture and to Mr Gordon McLachlin for his patience and encouragement over the past year.

My credentials are those of a sheltered life, no less than two-thirds of my professional career having been spent at the *BMJ*. After ten years of junior hospital posts in general medicine and pathology I started as an assistant editor and have remained at Tavistock Square, working in all sections of the journal as well as on specialist journals and books. I cherish in particular having worked under two great editors—Sir Theodore Fox of the *Lancet* (whom I encountered in a six month interlude during my house jobs) and Dr Hugh Clegg, editor of the *BMJ* for my first two years. In their case the judgment of history seems likely to repeat itself: just as Thomas Wakley, the charismatic founder of the *Lancet*, is remembered at the expense of the equally influential Ernest Hart at the *BMJ*, so I suspect that history will place Robbie Fox (happily still alive) above his contemporary at the *BMJ*, if only for the additional merit of being a delightful public figure and a witty speaker.

Both Fox and Clegg were powerful influences at an important time for British medicine; their different ways of working showed me that there are several paths to the same destination. Fox used outside assessment comparatively little and his own knowledge and insights a lot (though he thought deeply about the issues, as shown in his Heath-Clark lectures for 1963 (3)). Clegg insisted on peer review for any serious article, and together with (Sir Austin) Bradford Hill established criteria for assessing the statistical aspects of a paper.

Both editors had in common the ability to concede that their decisions might have been wrong and that they should take a fresh look at and advice about an article. In particular, I learnt from both that authors might well be justified in their complaints about whimsical, lazy, or incompetent evaluations and that an editor has two important roles *vis-a-vis* the author. Firstly, he should act as an ombudsman, protecting him from any unfairness by the referee. Second, the editor should play a part as a teacher, helping the author to improve both the scientific aspects and the presentation of his articles.

A further factor influencing my choice of topic was that I could pay tribute to a remarkable man and a remarkable institution. I met Franz Ingelfinger on only two or three occasions and wish it could have been more often. De Tocqueville commented that the special characteristic of the New Englanders was their ability to create voluntary bodies to achieve public purposes (4), and certainly Ingelfinger's journal, the *New England Journal of Medicine*, was, and continues to be, the finest general medical publication in the world, reflecting the curious blend of razor-sharp intellect and Bostonian common sense that is the hallmark of Harvard and its neighbouring medical institutions.

Among other things, Franz thought deeply and wrote lucidly about the problems of medical editing, a practice which his successor, Arnold Relman, and his deputy editors have continued and enhanced, as witness the many references by them in this monograph. In entitling my Rock Carling lecture 'A difficult balance: editorial peer review in medicine' I can pay tribute to one of Ingelfinger's most influential contributions, 'Peer Review in Biomedical Publication' (2). He started the debate which I shall be continuing, asking two fundamental questions: is validation really secured by the conventional system of manuscript review, and if so, is it worth the price? Even if I cannot wholly answer either of these, I hope to come up with some questions of my own.

Finally I should thank the principal people who helped me. My original interest in research into peer review was encouraged by Professor Hugh Dudley, who was never too busy to let me try out ideas, however *jejune*, on him and also made pithy comments on the manuscript; his colleague, Professor Andrew Nicolaides wrote the computer program for the study described in chapter 5 and helped over many of the statistical aspects, as did Professor David Barker, Professor Martin Gardner, Dr Selwyn St Leger, and Mrs Julie Morris. To Professor Rudolf Klein I owe a big debt for encouraging me when I was at a particularly low ebb of the study and pointing to some interesting parallels between editorial peer review and evaluations in the larger world. Professor Tony Mitchell helped me to sharpen some ideas at an early stage by organizing a public meeting for authors, referees, and editors at Nottingham in 1982. Dr Patricia Woolf, one of the pioneers in the study of piracy, plagiarism, and forgery, produced several new concepts, which have led to fascinating (and sometimes unrepeatable) discussions and conclusions.

Many people helped by answering queries on specific points or providing me with unknown references, or both: Dr Philip Altman, Professor David Apirion, Ms Kathy Case, Professor D. E. Chubin, Professor Stephen Cole, Dr B. C. Dodd, Dr Bernard Freedman, Dr Eugene Garfield, Dr Malcolm Godfrey, Professor T. Gustafson, Professor Marcel La Follette, Dr John Maddox, Professor J. L. Melnick, the Science Policy Research Unit, University of Sussex, Dr English Showalter, Mr Henry G. Small, Ms Jacqueline Stiles, Dr T. P. Stossel, Professor T. P. Whitehead, Dr P. O. Williams, and Professor Alfred Yankauer.

My fellow editors in the Vancouver Group and the BMA specialty journals answered questionnaires about semantics and helped me in numerous other ways. Dr Robert Burchfield, editor of the *Oxford English Dictionary*, was kindness itself in advising me about definitions, as was his colleague Mr A. M. Hughes (and almost all of the quotations in the chapter headings are taken from the *OED*.) No fewer than ten people read through the entire manuscript, three of the *BMJ* Smiths (Jane, Richard, and Tony) and Professor John Bailar, Sir Douglas Black, Professor Hugh Dudley, Dr David Evered, Dr Alex Paton, Professor Philip Rhodes, and Dr William Whimster.

Much of this monograph was written while I was a Rockefeller Scholar at that ideal place for tranquillity and work, the Villa Serbelloni in Bellagio, Italy. I am grateful to Professor Leonard Bruce-Chwatt for suggesting the possibility of going there and to its resident administrators, Dr Roberto Celli and Ms Angela Barmlettler, for their many kindnesses and for maintaining the genius of the place. Dr Kenneth Warren, who is the director for health sciences in the Rockefeller Foundation, has been a constant source of ideas and encouragement over several years, and I have made full use of his writings.

Finally, anyone who looks at the faces of my colleagues at the *BMJ* will perceive how much more strain I have thrown on them; in particular, I should like to thank Mr Derek Virtue for redrawing the illustrations, Ms Ruth Holland for all her help over the manuscript and in many other ways, Ms Ann Shannon for providing me with seemingly unobtainable references so speedily, and Ms Jane Smith, who has been a constant source of stimulation at all stages of the study and of writing the monograph.

1

Introduction

For several centuries science has grown at a steady and continuous rate. Half the scientists who have ever lived are alive today and the growth in their number has been matched by the growth in the number and variety of the scientific journals in which they publish their research. Yet, we might ask with Kingsley Amis whether such growth has been accompanied by a maintenance of standards: does 'more mean worse?'

There are still relatively few 'core' journals, which have wide readerships and publish important articles, and these can accept only a fraction of the articles submitted to them. The remainder find their way into a wide variety of journals, where many of them attract little attention. The authors of these neglected articles complain that they have been excluded unfairly from the core journals. The editors reply that they have made their choices in a way that is traditionally fair and rigorous—through peer review: submitting articles to outside experts for opinions on their merits.

Scientific facts and theories must survive critical study and testing by other competent and disinterested people, and publication plays a key part in this. Before the development of printing scientists communicated with each other by letters. Because of the possibilities for piracy they kept their findings to a small circle, with the obvious risk of a delay in or a lack of public recognition. Even after printing was established, scientists were still secretive about their work, and one of the concerns of the new scientific societies and academies of the seventeenth century was to encourage them to abandon this attitude (5).

References begin on p. 152

1

A major way of persuading them to do this was to ensure priority (giving the date on which the manuscript was first received); another was prompt publication together with an emphasis on the archival importance of the society's journal. Yet another was to ensure validation through scrutiny of the article before publication by representatives of a prestigious organization such as the Royal Society. Thus its *Philosophical Transactions* (begun in 1665, five years after its foundation) gradually began to distinguish between evaluated and unevaluated work.

By 1702 another major journal, the *Journal de Sçavans*, founded just before the Royal Society's *Transactions*, had assigned responsibility for the various disciplines to different members of the editorial board, which met regularly to discuss articles. Though peer review had its ups and downs for the next two centuries, it came to be used increasingly. Thus in the middle of the eighteenth century a President of the Royal Society, the Earl of Macclesfield, reminded the fellows that only through external scrutiny could suitable standards be maintained, and he set up a committee to do this.

Later, in 1796, such scrutiny was to lead the President, Sir Joseph Banks, to reject Jenner's account of the first use of vaccination against smallpox (6). Banks sent this to his friend, Sir Everard Home, for an opinion, who replied saying that he 'wanted faith'—in other words, the recommendations made from a study of one patient were not securely based. If 20 or 30 children were innoculated with the cowpox and afterwards for the smallpox without contracting the latter he might be led to change his opinion. Banks rejected Jenner's article for publication without sending it to the editorial committee, and Jenner then published his findings himself as a monograph. In this way the Royal Society was never associated with one of the most important medical discoveries of the eighteenth century even though it was made by one of its own fellows.

Much of this account is taken from an essay by Zuckerman and Merton (5), who seem also to have been the first to quote the now often-cited letter by Thomas Huxley.

Introduction

You have no idea of the intrigues that go on in this blessed world of science. Science is, I fear, no purer than any other region of human activity; though it should be. Merit alone is very little good; it must be backed up by tact and knowledge of the world to do very much.

For instance, I know that the paper I have just sent in [to the Royal Society] is very original and of some importance, and I am equally sure that if it is referred to the judgement of my particular friend . . . that it will not be published. He won't be able to say a word against it, but he will pooh-pooh it to a dead certainty.

You will ask with some wonderment, Why? Because for the last twenty years . . . has been regarded as the great authority on these matters, and has had no one to tread on his heels, until at last, I think, he has come to look upon the Natural World as his special preserve, and no poachers allowed. So I must manouevre a little to get my poor memoir kept out of his hands.

We also know that during his thirty years as editor of the *BMJ* from 1868 to 1898 Ernest Hart was regularly sending articles for external critical opinions. Conversely, the editors of the 'one man' journals, such as *Hoppe-Seylers Zeitschrift* and *Virchow's Archiv*, still decided themselves on which articles should be published—and even as recently as the 1960s the then editor of *Nature* is said to have relied mainly on expert opinions within the editorial office, taking the occasional article with him to ask a colleague's opinion over lunch at his London club.

By the end of the second world war, however, peer review was in large-scale use, being introduced, for example, by the *Journal of Clinical Investigation* in 1942 (7). Today it is practised all over the world: in the West at least three-quarters of the major scientific journals use peer review for assessing original articles for publication. In the USSR Relman found that the 100 medical journals were edited in much the same way as their American counterparts, with peer review of articles by members of the editorial boards and outside consultants; the reviews were mostly unsigned and the final decision about publication was taken by a vote of the editorial board (8). Most articles submitted for publication to the Chinese medical journals undergo peer review by two assessors, with a final rejection rate of about 75 per cent (Sun, presentation to the FIPP/WHO seminar in Copenhagen, November 1984).

Peer review is also, I hope to show, a microcosm of medicine and science in general. Such weighing in the balance may be for either high-flown purposes or mundane ones. For example, it may authenticate the substance of scientific work submitted for publication, thereby enabling an organization such as the Royal Society to maintain its authoritative status (5). Alternatively, it may be used for judging job applicants, competing claims for research grants, or which citations to use in a review article. Editors and their advisers make up one of the so-called gatekeepers of science (9), judges whose key role is to protect and enhance its norms. How competent are such judgments? Does peer review, in which outside experts are asked for their advice, achieve better results than editorial discretion by itself? How much does it delay publication, and can it be shown to improve articles? Can the dangers of timidity, bias, and caprice be abolished or appreciably diminished? Does peer review serve to accelerate or retard the progress of science? And what do the process and the outcome of such judgments tell us about the nature of science itself?

To try to answer some of these questions this book traces a path from present day practice to possible future developments. After looking at current methods of evaluating articles it examines the charges against peer review as well as the suggestion that it is essential for maintaining scientific standards, and concludes by proposing some improvements.

Inevitably much of this is based on my own experience of judgments as seen in a general weekly medical journal, which like most others receives far more submitted articles than it can ever print. The journal uses advice from outside experts on the merits of these articles as an important (but not the sole) factor in the decision whether to publish or not. Nevertheless, the results of my own research and the reviews of other surveys will inevitably impinge on wider issues, particularly the assessment of research before it is done—that is, applications for grants.

Introduction

Given the small amount of research that has been done into this topic, I shall have to draw on the experience of peer review in disciplines outside medicine, but, save in one or two details, there seems to be little difference in the practices and principles. I shall also draw on a study of my own, which aimed at answering some of these questions. The question that we have to answer, then, is how does peer review act for scientific journals: as a filter, preventing the publication of some articles altogether; or as a traffic policeman, directing articles away from some journals towards others? A further analogy to examine is whether the mass of journals acts as a sponge, ensuring that with persistence eventually no article remains unpublished; in this case peer review would act as a delaying device, but finally have no effect in preventing publication.

The answers to such questions may not be comfortable, but they are important. As I hope to show, the investment of time and money in peer review is high and the belief in its efficacy considerable. If these were unjustified then drastic improvements in peer review or its replacement by a totally different system would be an urgent priority for the scientific community.

2
Triage: the editorial process

Triage. (1717). *The action of sorting according to quality.*

Scientific journals have several functions: to inform, instruct, comment, and, possibly, amuse. Most of any major journal that is not devoted to reviews, however, must be taken up with original articles reporting advances in science. Here above all the editor is concerned to ensure quality, however this is defined, and much of this book is devoted to this problem.

Authors of articles are entitled to expect a consistent response from the editor: prompt and courteous treatment of their articles—and, since most editors and expert referees get a thrill from reading articles (not to mention being authors themselves), authors are likely to be treated in this way. They may also reasonably question why a paper has been turned down and ask the editor to consider it again. Here I explain how editors go about sorting original articles and the inherent difficulties.

Initially the editor carries out triage: classifying articles into self-evident masterpieces, obvious rubbish, and the remainder (usually the majority) needing careful consideration. It is in this last category that peer review plays such an important part.

When an article is sent to a journal it is first registered. This process records details such as the length, number of authors, copies, illustrations, and tables. The editor reads through the article to decide whether it deserves peer review. If so, he next decides which referee to send it to and, apart from the general questions asked about every article, what specific points need to be answered. Many journals use two external referees, either simultaneously or sequentially, though sometimes the editor or a member of his board is the

References begin on p. 152

second expert reader. Referees may be sent a form and asked to comment under particular headings (usually including a section for general remarks) or asked to answer a series of questions posed in the editor's letter. These include: are the findings original, for the world or the region (and if not, does their importance outweigh this consideration); are they scientifically reliable (including the methods, statistics, and deductions); and are they important for the readers of this journal?

CHOICE OF REFEREES

The choice of referees is not as haphazard as some people think: they may be acknowledged experts in the specialty or known to be doing research into a particular topic; they may be members of the editorial board or part of a larger group of advisers the journal uses regularly; they may be unknown but recommended by members of the board or the group of advisers; they may be known from their authorship or important articles on the subject.

Today many editorial offices have their referees listed on a card index or a computer; this enables greater selectivity, matching a referee to an article more closely than was possible in the past, not overloading him with too many requests, and also monitoring his performance (including the time he takes and the quality of his report). I believe that some such system is likely to be fairer than the former happy go lucky practice of picking a referee out of one's memory: it ensures that a journal uses less well-known assessors whose opinions cannot be 'guaranteed' in advance. True, there is the opposite argument: that an editor should choose an adviser whose biases and proclivities are well known to him. To my mind, however, such a practice has the risk of creating a charmed circle of referees whose opinions the editor can predict and can therefore determine the fate of any article from the start. There is no substitute for constantly striving to find new assessors.

In using outside assessors we at the *BMJ* follow similar policies and practices to those of other scientific editors.

7

Firstly, the referee is a specialist adviser and not the final decision maker. Second, we try to ensure fair and unbiased assessment of the article. Third, we try to explain our reasons for rejecting the article. Fourth, we tell the referee of our decision, particularly explaining any reasons for not following his advice.

GENERAL QUESTIONS

The general questions we ask about an article submitted to the *BMJ* concern its originality, scientific reliability, clinical importance, and suitability for our general journal as opposed to a specialist one. Other journals use a longer list with these questions as well as others (p. 110) (10) or with specific queries related to the discipline. We ask referees to be prompt, by returning the manuscript within two weeks; other editors are less insistent on speed and allow them up to two months.

Once the referee's reports are back, an editor can decide whether to accept the article as it stands, reject it outright, or consider it further. The last category includes several possibilities. Two referees may have produced totally opposite opinions and the advice of a third may be needed, to say who is more likely to be 'right' or to give another opinion about the article's merits.

One referee may not feel competent to judge part of the article—say, the statistical or biochemical aspects—and the editor may have to seek further advice. The referees may report that important details of the methods or the data are lacking from the paper, which should be reconsidered once these have been provided. The editor may think that the article is too long or obscure or has been aimed at the wrong readership and offer to consider a version revised to specific suggestions.

In all this the editor may be helped by an editorial committee. By analogy with the Royal Academy's selection panel, we call our editorial committee for the *BMJ* the 'hanging committee'. It meets weekly and is composed of two outside consultants (who change regularly, so they do not become part of a cosy coterie) and three members of the medical staff. Not only does the hanging committee read any article thought by an editor and the referee to be potentially suitable for publication: it also considers appeals from authors and holds general discussions on policy.

In practice, like many other journals we accept few articles for publication without asking the author to make some changes, however slight. For those that we do not accept the amount of information we give in the letter of rejection varies considerably. At one extreme, we return an article with a printed rejection slip or duplicated letter (as in poor quality or highly specialist articles); at the other extreme, we send a long letter of commentary together with detailed criticisms by one or two assessors. Again, when challenged by the authors, usually, like many editors, we seek advice from new assessors, asking them either to review the articles as new or to adjudicate between the original referee's opinions and the author's riposte. The older among us have always called this a judgment of Paris, but there is now a movement in the office to be pedantic and to ascribe it to Solomon. Perhaps neither the modern task nor the verdict is up to its ancient counterparts but the new assessor seems to enjoy his temporary role. Finally, a few editors will always insist that the original decision is final and is not open to appeal (11).

DELAY IN PUBLICATION

Authors often complain that the time spent delays the transmission of knowledge. Editors argue that time used in refining an article is well spent and is small compared with the time spent in research, writing it up, and unexplained delays. Thus, for 103 articles, written by authors from the Mayo Clinic, the time spent by the article in the editorial office was a small proportion of the total time from the origin of the idea to the final publication (figure 1) (12). Ingelfinger confirmed the lengthy interval between beginning a study and publication, finding that this varied

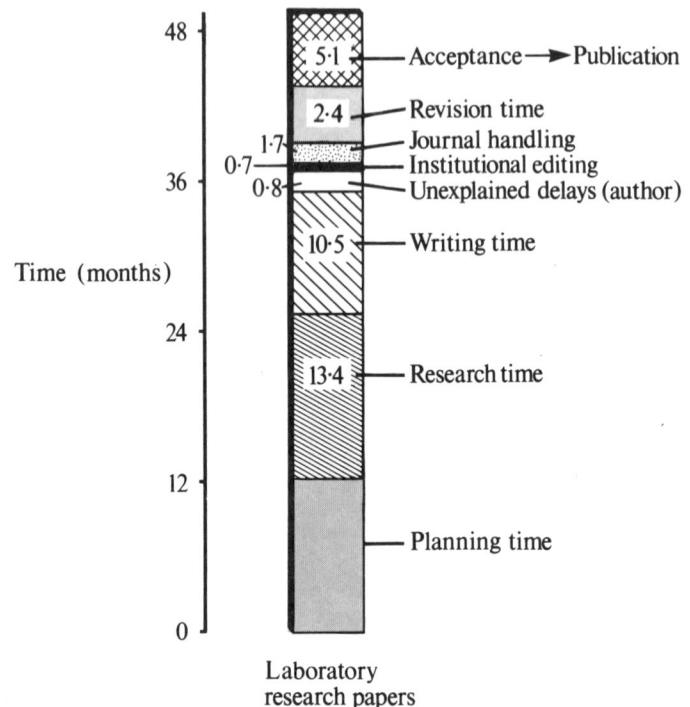

FIGURE 1. Components of time lapse between hypothesis and publication. (Reproduced, modified, from Roland and Kirkpatrick (12) by kind permission of the authors and the *New England Journal of Medicine*.)

according to the discipline: for the physical sciences it was 25 months, for social sciences 30 months, and for medical sciences 47 months (13). I have no data for this type of delay, but the delay in the office for an article submitted to the *BMJ* is short: a median of five weeks from receipt of an article to writing to the author with our decision. The median time to publication from receiving the corrected script is 10 weeks; any delay is usually due to the authors' failure to revise the text promptly.

Some authors still argue that such delays are too long, but a large proportion of workers in the specialty (possibly 60 per cent) (14) know of the findings well before they are

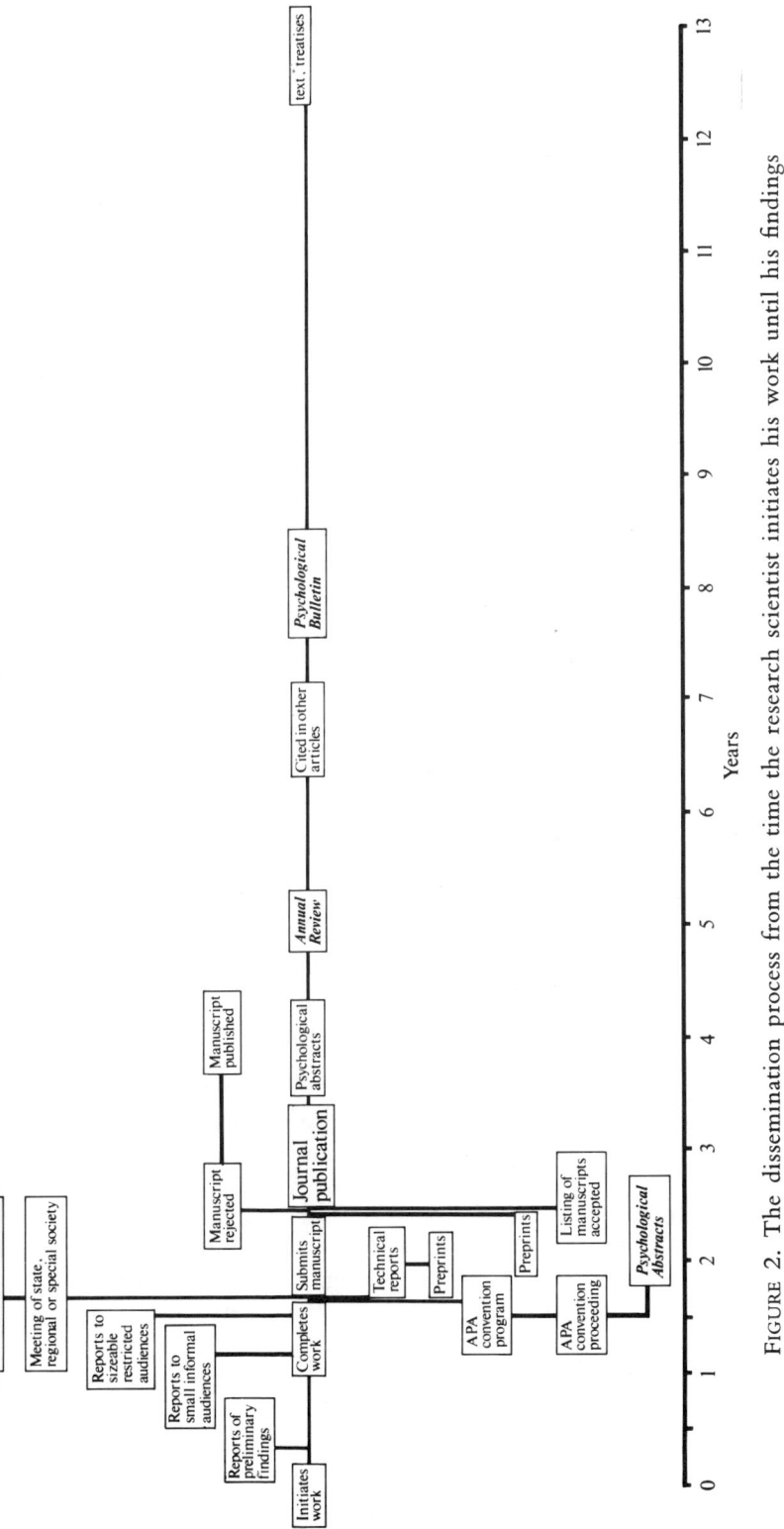

FIGURE 2. The dissemination process from the time the research scientist initiates his work until his findings become integrated into the fund of scientific knowledge. The abcissa gives the median time, after initiation of work, of each form of dissemination shown in the figure. (Reproduced, modified, from Garvey (16) by kind permission of the authors and publishers.)

published. In this, De Solla Price emphasized the role of the 'invisible colleges' (an elegant tribute to the name of the organization which preceded the formation of the Royal Society)—letters, assessing articles for publication, conversations, workshops, discussions at meetings, and preliminary presentations at conferences (15).

Each of the invisible colleges is concerned with research into a subset of knowledge, and they have an important role in propagating ideas—witness the striking prevalance in publications of allusions to informal communication. Thus 84 per cent of papers on cyclic adenosine monophosphate (cAMP) mentioned such personal communications (14), and before publication 61 per cent of scientists usually knew of the work described, and 13 per cent sometimes knew, often because of an association with a key figure, such as a leading research worker or a referee for the *Journal of Biological Chemistry*. On the other hand, most invisible colleges are made up of superspecialists, and scientists working elsewhere in the discipline may not know of these findings. For this reason, publication is vital in keeping them in touch with the important developments and enabling them to assess in detail the claims made.

Even after publication recognition may be slow (figure 2) (16). Depending on the subject, the first written mention (citation) of an article varies from an average of 18 months (physics) to 30 months (psychology). In microbiology the delay between the publication of an article and of an abstract varies from two weeks to 22 months (*Current Contents* being the quickest abstracting journal, with a median delay of $2 \cdot 5$ months) (17). Nevertheless, in developing countries an abstracting journal summarizing an article may arrive before the journal containing the primary publication—and in India, for example, the delay in the delivery of a journal published in the West is often similar to the delay between receipt and publication of the article (18). Finally, enshrinement as a fundamental reference may take as long as 10 years (though, conversely, in some subjects, particularly physics, the work is likely to have been long superseded by this time) (19).

CITATION ANALYSIS

Increasingly these days citations are being used to try to measure the pattern of the growth of science and to suggest its quality. These attempts have given rise to the discipline of citation analysis, though this has been going on for longer than most of us realize.

The first attempt at publication analysis goes back to 1917, for anatomy. The authors of this article recognized the difficulties as well as the promise, pointing out that, on the basis of figures alone, the author of many small ephemeral articles would be judged as of greater importance than, say, William Harvey, who had contributed just two works, though these were of great significance (20).

Citation analysis began properly in 1927 but was given its modern form in 1964 with the publication of Garfield's *Science Citation Index* (21). As well as enabling a reader to search through the relevant literature using references cited and citing references as a link between related papers, the *SCI* publishes figures for the number of citations an article receives in any year. It also publishes an impact factor for each journal, based on the number of citations received by articles it publishes. Since a few journals publish a large number of articles, using the number as an index of quality might overestimate their importance. If the total number of citations to the journal is divided by the total number of citable articles the journal printed that year, this 'impact factor' will help to correct any false impression.

Considerable claims have been made for the value of citation analysis in assessing the merits of scientists, journals, and articles. The majority of all references cite papers published in relatively few journals: only 25 journals are cited in 24 per cent of all references and only 125 journals in 50 per cent of all references. Only 540 journals are cited 1000 times or more a year. As a result, Garfield claims, it is possible to devise a multidisciplinary core for all science comprising no more than 1000 journals.

These claims have not gone unchallenged, and the debate goes on; one sensible conclusion seems to be that citation analysis is best used with other measures of quality.

Nevertheless, certain facts have been established beyond dispute. Top rank scientists (say, Nobel prize winners) publish more articles than lower rank scientists, in journals with high impact factors; most citations are not self-citations or negative comments rebutting the claims made in the cited article (22). The articles most often cited are not those primarily about methods but those about theories. Finally a small proportion of journals have much higher impact factors than others, and these are correspondingly more important in communication among research workers.

VARIATIONS ON EDITORIAL THEMES

There are many variations on these editorial arrangements. The pattern I have outlined has been nicely compared to an absolute monarchy: the Sun King (the autocratic chief editor) is in control, with a panel of referees and a board of members who meet once a year or less. The board members usually help to determine policy, monitor standards, and act as principal referees or adjudicators in disputes. Some general journals, such as the *BMJ* and the *New England Journal of Medicine*, have a 'hanging committee', which is particularly concerned with selecting articles for publication from a short list, and meets regularly, often once a week.

In another pattern the editor functions as a president, overseeing section editors, who deal with authors and referees. In a third pattern there is a co-operative, with all the editors having equal status and working independently together with an administrator, who may be an editor or a secretary (23). Most editors try to ensure that their editorial boards are broadly based, representing, say, all aspects of the discipline, academic and service interests, and the various parts of a country or region.

The second variation is in the use of outside referees. Some journals use these very little or not at all: in the latter category Virchow judged the articles himself, maintaining that anybody was free to make a fool of himself in the pages of *Virchow's Archiv* (24); the initial success of the *American Journal of Medicine* owed much to the encyclopaedic knowledge of its first editor, Alexander Gutman, who decided himself, usually within a couple of weeks, whether to accept a paper for publication (2); and until a few years ago the *Lancet* relied on in-house judgments for its decisions (25). But now this practice is unusual, and, at the other extreme, some journals regularly use more than two assessors: three is not uncommon (26), and *Current Anthropology* customarily solicits opinions from no fewer than 15 outside consultants, its editor maintaining that this is the only way to achieve fairness in a discipline that is riddled with controversy (27).

Thirdly, should authors be known to the referee and vice versa? To try to avoid personal bias, some journals routinely try to 'blind' the referee to the authors' identities by removing the first sheet of an article containing their names before sending it for an opinion (28). Others suggest that authors should write their articles so that these contain no internal clues to their identities, such as acknowledgements or references to previous work (29). Most referees' reports are still sent anonymously to the authors, so that referees will not be identified with their opinions and get into personal arguments. Some journals now prefer their comments to be signed, however, or at least give the consultants an option of signing them (30). Many journals send unsigned copies of the referees' opinions to the authors, and a few, such as the *British Journal of Surgery*, also send signed copies of one referee's report to the other assessor and vice versa (Dudley, personal communication). All these aspects are discussed in more detail later in this book.

PUBLIC DISCLOSURES

This, then, is an outline of the editorial process today as it has evolved from its beginnings with the *Journal des Sçavans* or the *Philosophical Transactions of the Royal Society* (5). Probably about three-quarters of major scientific journals use some system of peer review (31), which should serve three objectives: prevent publication of bad work; improve scholarship—to see that the relevant literature is cited and

Table I. Royal Society guidelines for peer review.

---

1. Every paper submitted to the journal for publication should be refereed.

2. Referees are appointed by the Editor, and report to him.

3. The name of any Referee may only be disclosed to the Author by permission of or at the request of the Referee, with the Editor's agreement.

4. The Referee may not disclose the contents of a paper submitted to him, nor make use of these for his own scientific work before publication, without explicit permission of the Author, to whom the name of the Referee must then be disclosed.

5. The Referee's report should contain a definite recommendation concerning publication based upon a reasoned judgment of the general form and scientific contribution of the paper as a whole. He may recommend acceptance outright or subject to revision of certain sections along specified lines, or may propose that the paper be substantially rewritten to improve the presentation or to strengthen the scientific argument. The substance of all such critical comments should be communicated to the Author for action, to the eventual satisfaction of the Referee. But failure to accept the Referee's view on all minor points of criticism should not be a bar to publication.

6. No paper should be rejected on the adverse report of a single Referee.

7. In the case of conflicting opinions, the Editor may appoint further Referees or an Adjudicator who may read all communications between the Author and Referees (whose names need not be disclosed to him).

8. A definite procedure should be established for Editorial decision within a stated period.

---

discussed in relation to the new findings—and improve the language and presentation of data (32).

Given the importance of these outcomes well-informed discussion of the process has been sparse. In 1975 the Scientific Information Committee of the Royal Society put forward a set of guidelines for peer review (table 1) (33). Disagreeing strongly with at least three of these (2, 4, and 8), *Nature* was concerned that such guidelines suggested a move towards uniformity, whereas what was wanted was more openness and the preservation of diversity to allow individual scientists to make individual choices.

If journals were to state regularly what their policy was in handling manuscripts, the editorial continued, and the extent to which editorial discretion entered, prospective authors would know better how they stood, and it printed a brief statement about *Nature's* own editorial procedures (34). Similarly *Science* has recently printed two editorials about its editorial policy, stating that initially all manuscripts will be ranked by a reviewing editor on a scale from 10 to 1 (11). On this basis, 60 per cent of manuscripts will be returned to the authors within ten days, the remainder being sent for peer review, with an eventual 50 per cent chance of being published. One rule, the editor states, will accompany these new changes; no resubmissions. We follow a similar procedure at the *BMJ*: about half the manuscripts are sent for peer review and two-fifths of these are eventually accepted—but we do allow appeals against decisions.

Increased openness must include similar attempts by editors and others to publicize their policies and the results of audits of the editorial process (35). One analysis of the latter had already appeared four years before the Royal Society's guidelines, when Harriet Zuckerman and Robert Merton published their key article on patterns of evaluation in science. This dealt with the institutionalization, structure, and functions of the referee system (5).

Drawing on their study of the rejection rates of a sample of 83 journals in the humanities, the social and behavioural sciences, mathematics, and the biological, chemical, and physical sciences, Zuckermann and Merton showed that the more humanistically orientated the journal, the higher the rate of rejecting manuscripts for publication; the more experimentally and observationally orientated, with an emphasis on rigour of observation and analysis, the lower the rate of rejection. Thus the mean rejection rate for the three history journals was 90 per cent and for the 12 physics journals 24 per cent. Journals in the same discipline showed a similar gradation: for the 11 of the 12 physics journals reporting new research findings, the mean rejection rate was 24 per cent, with proportions varying between 17 per cent and 25 per cent; for the twelfth journal the rejection rate was 40 per cent, but this proved the general rule, because its articles were concerned primarily with the humanistic, pedagogical, historical, and social aspects of physics.

Much of the study by Zuckermann and Merton was concerned with the effect of status differences among referees and among authors and between referees and authors, and it is referred to frequently throughout the rest of this book. Another major researcher into this topic was Michael Gordon. He also based part of his research on archival material for physical sciences journals, but conducted a series of unstructured interviews with the editors of 32 research journals as well (36). He confirmed that journals in the physical, geophysical, and chemical sciences had the lowest rejection rates (10–37 per cent), with a hierarchy as follows: mathematical journals 50 per cent; specialist biomedical journals 45–67 per cent; social sciences journals 75–80 per cent; and philosophy journals 90 per cent. The anomalies in this pattern were the *BMJ* and the *Lancet*, with rejection rates of 80–85 per cent, but, given that both of these are general rather than specialist, this finding confirmed the general rule that, the more humanistically orientated a journal, the higher its rejection rate. Four of Gordon's sample of journals regularly used no external assessor, 17 used one, 7 used two, and for 4 the number varied between one and three.

A further survey of editorial process in the earth sciences was undertaken for a conference of editors in 1975 (31). Some 90 journals had editorial boards, and 58 did not; in 31 cases these met regularly to consider manuscripts. All papers were refereed in 91 out of 134 journals (compared with 61 out of 71 found in a similar survey for the life sciences (37)), the referees being selected by the editor in 69 cases, the editorial board in 22, and both in 12. In most cases the list of referees was larger than the editorial board, but only 30 out of 138 journals had an established list.

INDIVIDUAL JOURNAL AUDIT

Several accounts have discussed the broader aspects of the process or the outcome, or both, of peer review for individual journals. They show how much work is entailed at all levels. Some of these document only crude rejection rates: 90 per cent for the *New England Journal of Medicine* (38) and 66 per cent for the *Journal of Clinical Investigation* (which in 1973 used 1150 assessors from all over the world, many of them more than once) (7, 39).

An analysis of the reasons for the rejection of 600 manuscripts submitted to *Social Science Quarterly* in 1973 and 1976 showed the following: unimportant or insignificant 29 per cent, flawed methods 26 per cent, unsound theoretical framework 21 per cent, poor presentation 10 per cent, or failure to meet editors' criteria 13 per cent. In no case was a manuscript rejected for poor presentation alone (40).

In 1975 the *Journal of Endocrinology* used 365 referees to assess 306 full papers and 115 short communications, with two assessors per article; the respective rejection rates were 43–51 per cent and 35–40 per cent. Of 51 consecutive articles not one was acceptable as it stood and modifications were necessary in the 31 accepted. Of the rejections, 11 articles had unvalidated or unreliable methods, 18 were too long in relation to the subject, one was more appropriate to another journal, and one was rejected on ethical grounds (41).

1–2 per cent of articles submitted to the *American Journal of Diseases of Children* were simply unworthy of publication; 85 per cent of reviews were completed within four weeks, usually being detailed and thoughtful critiques. Though the editor took the decision to reject an article, for fairness he had an additional review by another referee first (42). For the 639 papers received by the *American Journal of Public Health* in 1979 the acceptance rate was less than 20 per cent; in about a third of cases the decision was made in the editorial office, either by the editor alone or by the editor in conjunction with the editorial board, the remaining papers being sent out to two or more referees (43).

Of 500 papers submitted consecutively to the *Australian and New Zealand Journal of Psychiatry*, 426 were sent for peer review, usually by two consultants. The latter saw a mean of seven papers (range 1–27) between April 1978 and July 1983; initially 18 per cent of papers were accepted and 33 per cent rejected, revision being suggested in 48 per cent of cases before a decision could be taken (44).

How much work a full-scale peer review system can entail is illustrated by a report by the Publication Committee of the American Physical Society (45). The two journals *Physical Review* and *Physical Review Letters* have a computerized file of 10,000 assessors. In 1979–80 about half of these were asked to assess one or more manuscripts: 1300 assessors received a single paper for review, but the 100 busiest referees (many of them members of an editorial advisory board) each received 10. Between a third and a half of the articles were seen by one assessor, the remaining papers requiring two or more referees' reports.

Finally, the editors of the BMA specialty journals produce excellent reports for the annual meetings of their editorial boards, an outstanding one being that for *Thorax*, whose editor has allowed me to quote some of his findings for 1984. With a circulation of 4000 copies, *Thorax* received 564 articles for publication in 1983–84, of which 203 were accepted. For surgical papers the mean interval from submission to verdict was 34 days (range 0–77) and for medical ones the median was 34 days (range 0–97); the interval between acceptance and publication was 4 months. In this year for the first time half the papers were assessed by two referees, with four major effects; it increased the editorial workload; it increased the work of the editorial board, each member of which on average saw 16 papers in the year; it increased the participation of other assessors (209 of whom were used); and it increased the mean submission to verdict interval, since a judgment of Paris (Solomon) had to be obtained when the two disagreed (the pattern being shown in figure 3).

Clearly, with the many thousands of refereed journals, the costs of peer review (in terms of both time and money)

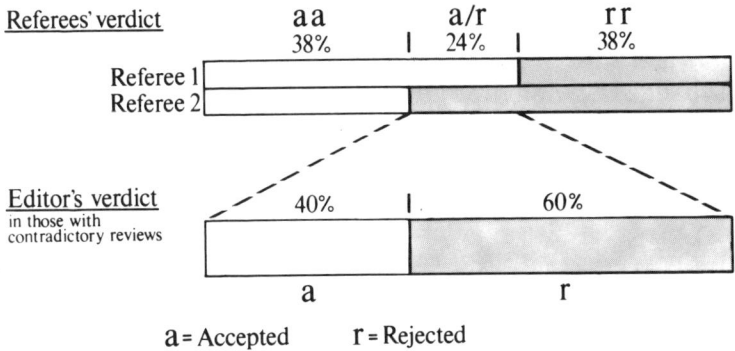

Referees' verdict

a a 38% | a/r 24% | r r 38%

Referee 1
Referee 2

Editor's verdict
in those with
contradictory reviews

40% | 60%

a   r

a = Accepted   r = Rejected

FIGURE 3. Consensus between referees' and editors' judgment. (Reproduced by kind permission of Dr Alistair Brewis, editor of *Thorax*.)

must be enormous, a theme I shall return to for medical journals in the next chapter. The original reasons for introducing peer review still obtain: as producers, scientists want to have their work protected (to avoid 'philosophicall robbery' (as Robert Boyle called plagiarism)), validated, and then published to their peers, and, as consumers, they want to be assured that the work of others is authentic (5). Even more than before, editors feel unable to judge the quality of highly specialist papers without expert help. Moreover, we now ask even more of peer review than this, while peer review has been applied to other problems, particularly applications for research funding.

With the power of such a system, not to mention the emotions evoked by it, it would be surprising if a vast number of objections had not been raised over the past 300 years to both the principle and the practice. Some of these are obvious sour grapes; others raise fundamental questions demanding answers, which this book will try to provide. At opposite poles of opinion, we need to know whether we support Professor John Ziman: 'The referee is the lynchpin about which the whole business of science is pivoted' (46) or a former editor of a then largely unrefereed journal, the *Lancet*, Sir Theodore Fox, who wrote in his Heath Clark lectures: 'When I divide the week's contributions into two piles—one that we are going to publish and the other that we are going to return—I wonder whether it would make any real difference to the journal or its readers if I exchanged one pile for another' (3).

3

Blemishes I:
what's wrong with peer review?
—process

Blemish (1555). *A defect, imperfection, flaw, in any object, matter, condition, or work.*

Process (1887). *The continuing interaction of human groups and institutions especially as observed and studied through its effects in social, political, cultural, etc, life, with the aim of finding underlying patterns in the data available.*

Peer review is not cheap: in 1979 Relman estimated that every year for the *New England Journal of Medicine* it occupied six or seven man-years of work by assessors outside the editorial office and another two man-years for those within it (47). If only half of the 20,000 or so biomedical journals (as well as of the 100,000 science journals) use outside assessors, the load of refereeing must be enormous, particularly when added to the other outside commitments of many reviewers, such as refereeing research grant applications and serving on appointments committees.

Another aspect Relman estimated was financial cost: for about 2500 articles this was a total of $100,000, or $40 per article. Gordon also provided some costs of refereeing, estimating for 510 articles reviewed for two hours each by a referee that the minimum direct costs were £2740, or over £5 per article at 1976 prices; adding in direct cost as well, including expenditure by the host institutions of the editors and referees (with an allowance for their salaries), more than doubled these (36).

Finally, I have estimated the cost of peer review for each article submitted to the *BMJ* in 1984 as at least £48 (details in table II), given that 1886 articles were refereed and that

References begin on p. 154

Table II. Costs of peer review (1984).

	£
Salaries (the equivalent of two medical editors and two secretaries working full time: members of hanging committee; and statistical advisers)	180,000
Office costs	10,000
Referees (1880 at £10 each)	18,800
Postage	2500
	£211,300

A total of 4431 new original articles was considered in the year
∴ cost of peer review per article=£211,300÷4431≃£48

reviewing occupied the equivalent of the time of two full-time medical editors and their secretaries; other payments were made to the expert assessors (usually a notional £10 for each article reviewed), statistical advisers, and members of the hanging committee.

Can we justify these costs by showing that peer review is 'worth it'—drawing up a balance sheet between the known costs and the advantages? If we could show, say, that peer review prevented the publication of unoriginal or unscientific articles, then we could decide whether the ends justified the means. Unfortunately, our measurements are inadequate, but we have a few facts relating to both process and outcome. The remainder of this chapter will consider the first of these.

CONSENSUS

One important aspect of the process is how far two assessors agree about an article. This consensus varies according to the discipline, Zuckermann and Merton finding that it was high in physics, two referees agreeing on a recommendation in 167 out of 172 papers evaluated for the *Physical Review* (5). For the social sciences, referees agreed on acceptance or rejection in 73 per cent of 193 original articles submitted to the *American Sociologist*, compared with 54 per cent expected by chance, and for 1572 articles submitted to two unnamed biomedical journals consensus was 75 per cent, compared with 62 per cent expected by chance.

Though he did not give the statistical methods used, or

the consensus level expected by chance, Ingelfinger's experience at the *New England Journal of Medicine* was the same; indeed, the 41 per cent perfect consensus came about chiefly because both reviewers graded a quarter of the 496 papers as D, or poor (2). For the *American Journal of Public Health* (43) there was 57 per cent complete agreement and 9 per cent complete disagreement for about 400 articles reviewed by two assessors. Finally, there was a consensus of 80 per cent between two reviewers for 249 papers accepted by the *IRCS Journal of Medical Science* (36).

Thus apparently more experts disagree about articles submitted to biomedical journals than they do about others. I will instance some possible reasons for this in describing my own prospective study of 1551 articles submitted to the *BMJ* (chapter 5). But at this point in discussing the peer review process a large spanner must be thrown into the works: a provocative study by two psychologists, Douglas Peters and Stephen Ceci (48,49).

This study may be neither the largest nor the most rigorous of those on peer review, but it has provoked the most discussion for several reasons. Firstly, the journal that eventually published their article accompanied it by commentaries invited from 59 experts. Second, the facts appeared under various guises at various times (50,51). Third, the whole conflation of original findings, arguments, editorial commentary, and ripostes adds up to what many scientists still believe: peer review is incompetent; heavily biased by factors such as personal and institutional status, sex, and nationality; and open to abuse because of research conflicts of interests between the author and the referee. (A further possible conflict of interest has been suggested recently—financial.)

In the 1970s Peters and Ceci took a broad sample of 13 influential psychological journals all with high impact factors and rejection rates (80 per cent). They chose at random one article from each journal with an author from a high prestige institution (defined by the research grant allocation) published in the previous 18–32 months; these had obtained above average citations.

Peters and Ceci altered the articles in several ways: they changed the names, but not the sex, of the authors; they changed the authors' institutions to fictitious ones—for example, the Tri-Valley Center for Human Potential; and they made slight ('cosmetic') alterations to the titles, abstracts, and opening paragraphs of the introductions. They then resubmitted the revised articles to the journals that had originally published them. Peters and Ceci did not tell the editors and referees about the study until the resubmission was detected or until the study was finished, but they did obtain permission from the authors. They did not name the journals concerned in their article.

One article had to be excluded from the study because the journal had changed its policy about the type of paper it accepted. Three articles were recognized as resubmissions of previously published work. The remaining nine out of the 12 manuscripts, however, were not detected as being unoriginal; one was accepted for publication and the remainder were rejected—not on grounds of unoriginality (which was not mentioned) but of poor study design, inadequate statistical analysis, and poor quality.

Given no obvious major shift in the journals' criteria for selecting referees, Peters and Ceci concluded that their findings might have two explanations. Firstly, the reviewers for the resubmitted article were less competent than for the original version, or, second, there was systematic bias towards the authors' institutions: an article from an ivy-leaf university would be treated more favourably than one from an unknown institution in Texas. The first possibility seems unlikely, but the question of bias (which Peters and Ceci believe explains their findings) needs to be examined.

BIAS

Personal

Authors often complain that assessors are biased against them on personal grounds. There is little objective evidence for this; rather the evidence is of 'positive' rather than 'negative' personal bias—in other words, decisions are biased in favour of known authors rather than against unknown ones. The rejection of the original paper on the first law of thermodynamics by the *Annales der Physik* in 1842 is often cited; its author, Karl Meyer, was a little known, modest postgraduate student and it was another 30 years before the importance of his article (published in a little known journal) was recognized (52). In science, early this century, a paper by several authors, with the well-known physicist Lord Rayleigh among them, was initially rejected for presentation at a meeting of the British Association for the Advancement of Science, only to be accepted after the authorities had been told that Rayleigh's name had inadvertently been left off the article (1).

This apparent preference for men of eminence is known as the 'halo' effect, or more popularly as the 'Matthew' effect, from Merton's famous essay in which he quotes the gospel: 'For whosoever hath, to him shall be given and he shall have more abundance; but whosoever hath not, from him shall be taken away even that he hath' (53). Accomplishments by those who are not yet famous tend to be underestimated, Merton suggests, later ones overestimated, particularly when they have won high distinctions, such as the Nobel Prize.

Such distinctions affect authorship: a Nobel laureate often wonders whether he should put his name on to articles; if he does, the articles are read, but he may be remembered wrongly as the only author; if he does not, the paper is read very little (between 15 and 23 per cent of readers chose which article to read according to the identity of the author (54)). In her book on Nobel laureates, *Scientific Elite*, Zuckermann showed that they tend to give first author place to co-authors (so-called noblesse oblige), and that those who become eminent before the prize transfer first authorship earlier than the less eminent future laureates. Both sets of authors increase noblesse oblige after getting the prize.

Status

The data on the referees' opinions and the editorial decision, then, support possible status bias rather than personal bias. In particular, the author's status may affect whether his article is sent for peer review at all and who is asked to assess it. Reviewing the archives of the *Physical Review*, containing 14,515 articles submitted between 1948 and 1956, Zuckermann and Merton classified their authors into three ranks: the first had won one of the most respected prizes or were members of prestigious societies, the second were listed in the archives of contemporary physicists, and the third were the remainder; there was also a large mobile subgroup (those who were changing from one rank to the next) (5).

The authors' rank was correlated with the mean number of papers they published over a year (4, 3·5, and 2, respectively, for top, medium, and lower ranks, with a very high mean figure of 15 for 47 per cent of the mobile subgroup). Rank was not correlated, however, with the number of articles the authors submitted to *Physical Review.* There was a considerable difference in the journal's acceptance rates, 91 per cent *v* 73 per cent for the top and bottom ranks, respectively.

The higher the rank of the author, the more frequently, Zuckermann and Merton found, did the editor of the *Physical Review* take a decision without using peer review (58, 73, and 87 per cent of papers from the three ranks were sent for external assessment). Reviewers were drawn disproportionately from the top rank: 5 per cent of authors but 12 per cent of referees were from this stratum—and these 12 per cent contributed to a third of all the judgments. Finally, 74 per cent of the authors and 45 per cent of the referees were aged under 40. There was no consistent pattern of allocation of referees to authors, the skill and competence of the former being the principal criteria. Most importantly, the relative status of the referee and the author had no influence on the recommendations on the article.

Gender

In a commentary on the paper by Peters and Ceci, Horrobin cites an unreferenced report that a number of women complained to the Modern Language Association of America that surprisingly few articles in the journal were by women.

Under pressure the association instituted a 'blind' reviewing procedure; thereafter the acceptance rate of papers by women rose dramatically.

In fact, the current executive director of the association, Dr English Showalter, wrote to me, the rate of acceptance of essays by women had risen well before the blind reviewing policy took effect in 1980, possibly related to the debates whether to institute blind reviewing or not. In 1963 ten of the 73 authors of published articles were women (14 per cent). From 1973 to 1982 some 80 of 280 authors of published articles were women (29 per cent); this period included the four years from 1973 to 1976 when the acceptance rate for articles written by men was almost twice as high as for those written by women. Since 1977 the rates have been virtually identical: 4·8 per cent for men, 4·4 per cent for women. Hence these changes may reflect the altered position of women in society in general rather than showing any bias towards gender; for the Modern Language Association of America the number of women in the senior editorial committees rose in this period, from two out of a total of 18 in 1973 to 17 out of 33 in 1985.

Institution

Zuckermann and Merton found that the assessors for the *Physical Review* were applying the same standards to papers whether they were written by junior or senior authors or had come from top-level institutions or otherwise. Thus reviewers from minor universities were no more likely to recommend acceptance of articles from minor universities than were reviewers from major universities. On the other hand, the thrust of the argument by Peters and Ceci was that the disguised articles had been rejected because of the lowered prestige of the authors' institutions: the first authors 'may have received a less critical, more benign evaluation than did our unknown authors from 'no-name' institutions'.

Other authorities are divided about this aspect. A young faculty member at the University of North Dakota in the 1960s was unable to publish 15–20 articles in mainstream psychological journals; after he had been at Harvard for a few years he had published most of these in the same journals (55).

In an experimental study the address of the author of an article was changed from a prestigious university to an unknown institution and then sent for peer review (56). Institutional prestige had no influence on the evaluation by 68 referees sent one version or the other. And, again for psychology, these findings have been confirmed: for 60 articles published in 1975 by the *Journal of Abnormal Psychology* the 1980 citation rates were 3·77 and 1·40 for authors from high and low status institutions respectively (57). This difference was significant, but it was comparable with the significant difference found for a second sample of papers published in another psychology journal where the referees had been blinded to the identity of the authors, who came from high or low status institutions.

So, given that the vast majority of published articles come from lower status institutions, is not the prestige of an institution one valid criterion in the editor's decision? No one could oppose this view provided status does not play a major part. After all, good workers tend to be at high status institutions because they are good; they have much more opportunity for informed comment from their colleagues, about both the proposed research and the resultant articles; and they have much more reputation to lose if they are shown consistently to publish bad work.

Research attitudes

One explanation for any institutional bias may be whether the assessors and authors have the same research attitudes. In a retrospective study of 2572 referees' reports on 1980 articles in two physical sciences journals, Gordon found that referees showed a preference for articles written by their own countrymen (table III). Referees from major universities showed a preference for articles coming from major universities; referees from minor universities, however, showed little preference for papers from either major or minor universities (table IV) (36). Hence, Gordon

Table III. Percentage of papers rated 'good' by referees.

	UK Authors	N. American Authors	Totals
UK Referees	70% of 600 papers	65% of 307 papers	907
N. American Referees	66% of 35 papers	75% of 20 papers	55
Total	635	327	962

Significance levels are limited, since the number of North American referees was so small, but UK authors were, on average, less critically evaluated by UK referees than they were by North American referees ($\chi^2=3\cdot365$), while North American authors were less critically evaluated by North American referees ($\chi^2=0\cdot8603$). Hence UK referees evaluated UK authors' papers less critically than they did those of North American authors ($\chi^2=2\cdot8584$) and North American referees evaluated North American authors' papers less critically than they did those of UK authors ($\chi^2=0\cdot7379$), So, while levels of significance are limited, a higher frequency of favourable evaluation of papers by co-nationals was indicated in each of the four possible cases.

(Reproduced from Gordon (36) by kind permission of the author and publishers.)

concluded, when referees and authors in the physical sciences are members of the same groups, whether national or institutional, the former are more likely to be less critical.

Support for Gordon's suggestion comes from an earlier analysis of some characteristics of authors and editors for three American journals: *American Sociological Review, American Economic Review*, and *Sociometry* (9). Two of these had used blind review over part of the study period, while the third had not. In the selection of articles for publication a more important influence than blind review was found to be the academic background (current affiliation and university giving doctorate) and the professional age of the editors (time since obtaining a doctorate): both of these were similar to those of the authors of published articles.

In the earlier period studied, most of the authors and the editors had received their doctorates from major universities. Hence any bias was linked with the common viewpoints based on training rather than on personal factors. This was supported by the finding that in the later

Table IV. Percentage of papers rated 'good' by referees.

	Minor University	Major University	Total
Minor University Referees	65% of 120 papers	67·5% of 80 papers	200
Major University Referees	50% of 110 papers	82·5% of 309 papers	419
Total	230	389	619

There is little difference between the frequencies with which minor university referees evaluated minor and major university authors' papers as 'good' ($\chi^2=0·13369$); but a massive difference between the frequencies with which major university referees favourably evaluated major and minor university papers ($\chi^2=44·585$).

Minor university authors were more frequently evaluated favourably (ie, less critically) by minor university referees ($\chi^2=5·295$), while major university authors were more often evaluated favourably by major university referees than they were by those affiliated to minor universities ($\chi^2=8·78$).

(Reproduced from Gordon (36) by kind permission of the author and publisher).

study period the academic backgrounds of the editors became more diverse and so did those of the contributors.

Obviously, then, shared viewpoints do play an important part in the referee's judgement, a fact emphasized by the experimental study already referred to (56). Some 67 reviews were obtained from 75 referees invited to assess a brief research article purportedly intended for publication in a symposium on 'Current Issues in Behaviour Modification'. All the papers had identical bibliography, introduction, and methods sections, and all were assessed blindly by the reviewers. The data section and the discussion were, however, altered either to conform to the referee's perspective (positive) or to oppose it (negative). In addition, some referees were asked to assess incomplete manuscripts without the results or discussion sections or both. (They were told that these sections were in preparation and that there was a strict deadline for publication.) The final five groups, which included another version of the article with 'mixed' results (both positive and negative), are shown in table V.

Table V. Study of assessors' reviews according to their perspectives.

Group	Results	Discussion
1	Positive	None
2	Negative	None
3	None	None
4	Mixed	Positive
5	Mixed	Negative

The assessors' views on the relevance of the topic studied were not affected by whether the papers were positive or negative, or incomplete. For the methods section, however, there was a statistically significant difference: reviewers rated a manuscript reporting positive results as methodologically better than one reporting negative results. The same differences were found for the reviewers' assessments of the presentation of data and of the article's overall scientific contribution. When the article was incomplete and contained no results the reviewers rated the manuscript much higher than when it contained them.

The results of this study are certainly provocative and I wonder whether they would apply to medicine, where the data tend to be more absolute and less easy to change so completely and convincingly. Much of the research into peer review has been concerned with sociology and psychology, disciplines where feelings run high and the existence of various schools of thought makes the attainment of a gold standard even harder than in medicine. What these findings do show for all disciplines is the necessity for choosing reviewers with different standpoints, both *vis-à-vis* the authors and one another, and for the editor to know these and to monitor how they affect decisions.

Conflicts of interest

If the editor should ensure that there are some conflicts of research interest between the author and the referee so as to achieve fully rounded opinions, he may nevertheless not know of personal antagonisms. All he can do is to monitor the recommendations, at the same time asking his assessors to declare any serious biases and to return the article if they find these overwhelming (see chapter 6).

Another aspect has recently been noted in the context of commercial interests and possible plagiarism (discussed more fully in the next chapter). More than once in 1983 the publication of an article in the *New England Journal of Medicine* caused sharp fluctuations in the stock market (58). The journal's policy remained that manuscripts should be selected for publication solely on grounds of merit and suitability, and its editor emphasized the value of disclosure. Authors should routinely acknowledge in a footnote all funding sources supporting the submitted work; other kinds of commercial associations should be volunteered in a covering letter to the editor, who, if he was going to accept the article, would then decide how much disclosure was necessary.

These proposals were supported in the subsequent correspondence (59—62), though one writer thought that they had not gone far enough: both reviewers and the editorial staff of medical journals should also declare any outside commercial interests (59), a suggestion that the *NEJM* had already partly acted on, in that the deputy and associate editors had filed disclosure statements (63)

The editor of *Nature* has also recently emphasized that an unpublished manuscript may have great financial as well as scientific value for the referee (64). The latter now often has links with some commercial organization, commonly undisclosed, and might take unfair advantage of privileged information in an article.

Commentators' criticisms

The next chapter discusses other features of peer review that are flawed. Here I shall finish discussing some aspects of the study by Peters and Ceci, though its themes run through this monograph as a *leit-motiv*, almost as obsessionally (to mix my metaphors) as the Suez canal ran through Lady Eden's drawing room during the 1956 Suez crisis.

Several of the commentators supported Peters' and Ceci's

conclusions about the dominant role of personal or institutional bias. Others were surprised by the findings, claiming that they reflected gross incompetence by the referees, and yet others criticized specific aspects of the study. Comments on this last category fall under three main headings: ethics, methods, and data analysis.

Ethics

One objection was to the ethics of the study, given that the editors and assessors had not been told about it until it was over. Thus one comment was that it had violated several of the ten ethical principles of the American Psychological Association (65), a claim countered by a list of many good points about it (66) and by the view, supported from the *Talmud*, that the benefits were potentially great since the research had gone to the heart of scientific endeavour (67). Nevertheless, these had to be balanced against the deception entailed, the extra time spent by editors and reviewers, and the ensuing discomfiture and embarassment. A balance sheet is shown in table VI.

Riposting, Peters and Ceci pointed out that, though seven commentators had criticized the ethics of deception, four had found it justified—as had by implication at least 11 others, who had encouraged Peters and Ceci to extend their study to other disciplines—and none of the editors or assessors of the two journals which had rejected their article (*Science* and *American Psychologist*) had commented on this aspect.

Believing that violation of a code of ethics could not occur in the abstract but must be seen in context, Peters and Ceci considered that cost-benefit analysis showed the deception to be warranted by the results, which no other method could have produced. I would support this view: the deception seems to me to be trivial and the results sufficiently important and provocative to warrant ruffling a few feathers.

Methods

Self-evidently, the sample of articles Peters and Ceci used was small and their methods were incomplete and open to

Table VI. Ethics of deception: cost–benefit analysis.

Non-commendable (Fleiss (65))	*Commendable* (Millman (66))
Possible violation of copyright law	Authors' and publishers' permission in most cases
Deception of editors and referees	Interesting question discussed
Unethical action of some editors in providing referees' comments	
	Good documentation about previous work
Possible identification of some authors	
	Good rationale for manipulating independent variable
	Good description of study
	Good methods (in disguising papers and lag between publication and resubmission)
	Plausible explanations and convergent and opposing evidence presented
	Implications discussed and suggestions made

question. For example, would the so-called 'slight' or 'minimal' changes have unfavourably impressed the second group of editors and reviewers, and what was the effect of the conversion of tables to graphs and vice versa? (68) Were, moreover, the fictitious names plausible and why did not the reviewers become suspicious of the mythical institutions and try to check on them? In fact, one claim was that the research design using fictitious institutional names ensured the conclusion, and it would have been better to have used lower ranking real institutions (69).

There was no evidence that both sets of reviewers had been comparable in demography, competence, or institutional status. Thus, the second set of reviewers might have come from more prestigious institutions; they would probably then have been more critical and wary of manuscripts, with more confidence in their own reviewing skills. A better design would have been to test a mixture of previously rejected or accepted and published articles from prestigious or non-prestigious institutions against a prestigious or non-prestigious resubmission.

Moreover, I believe that yet a further variable should have been added: the prestige of the journal, with articles in the study having been accepted or rejected by both prestigious or non-prestigious journals. In their riposte Peters and Ceci also suggested further controls (a final design, which is enough to put any editor off research, is shown in table VII).

Analysis

Several commentators observed that Peters and Ceci were confusing systematic bias with random error. Given that the journals' rejection rates were about 80 per cent, they might have obtained the same results if they had resubmitted the articles without altering the authors' affiliations (70). Even in a journal with a 45 per cent acceptance rate, such as *Physical Review Letters*, the chance of an article being accepted without any revisions was only 10–15 per cent (71). Thus if 25 per cent of the papers had been conspicuously bad, the proportion of acceptance among the nine unrecognized papers would have been 0·22; in fact it was 0·11, not significantly different at the 5 per cent level (72). Another writer made the point that the data suggested a positive bias in the first review and a negative one in the second (73).

One comment on the study's finding that seven out of eight pairs of reviewers agreed on rejection was that this was an unheard of level of reliability, with a kappa value of agreement of 1·0, compared with the highest value reported of 0·52 for the *American Psychologist* (74). Again, it was alleged that the literature review was selective, with some of it showing higher consensus than Peters and Ceci had stated; one study showed 79 per cent of reviewers substantially in agreement; another journal reported a kappa value of 0·49, much greater than would have been expected by chance alone (75). Nevertheless, Peters and Ceci argued that their

Table VII. Design of study controlling for variety of factors.

Author status (high v low) × author institution (prestigious, non-prestigious but real, fictitious) × reviewer status (high v low) × journal status (high v low) × scientific discipline (social science v physical science) × paper's history (published, rejected, new submission)

---

reporting was accurate and that in fact the 79 per cent figure was misleading since only 65 per cent of the reviewers agreed precisely.

Undoubtedly, then, the study by Peters and Ceci has many flaws, mainly inherent in its design, particularly the small numbers. Its great merit is that it has made everybody who has heard about it, whether authors, referees, or editors, stop and think about the issues. Any rigorous study to confirm or refute their findings would be inordinately costly and complicated. Given that some of the studies I have cited claim that consensus between two or more assessors is not much higher than chance, does their study and the studies by others suggest that the outcome is any better with peer review than it is without? In other words, does the system pick 'better' papers (as judged by citation analysis, among other things) than no system would—and in any case how can the process and the outcome of peer review be improved? These issues will be discussed in the subsequent chapters.

4

Blemishes II:
what's wrong with peer review?
—outcome

Outcome—'The subject of medical audit is at present
too much confined to journals . . . for its terminology to
have found its way into the [Oxford English
Dictionary's] files' (Hughes, personal communication).

In some ways assessing the outcome of editorial peer review
is easier than the process. To repeat the main questions (p.
5), do journals act as a sponge or a filter (76), or does peer
review act merely as a traffic policeman—and does it result
in revision of the articles? These questions may be answered
by looking at three features. Firstly, the fate of articles
rejected by a journal; are these published elsewhere and are
they cited? Second, the type of errors in articles published in
good quality journals that peer review has apparently failed
to identify. Third, deficiencies in the assessor's report.

FATE OF REJECTED ARTICLES

In a small-scale survey of a random sample of 300
manuscripts rejected by the *New England Journal of Medicine*
in 1975, some 85 per cent of the authors replying to a
questionnaire (with a 50 per cent response rate) said that
these had been published elsewhere—in other general
research, specialty, or state journals (47). Given that the
NEJM accepts only 12–15 per cent of articles, and that
there is an arbitrary element to the editorial process, some of
the publication in other prestigious journals might have
been predicted. Surprisingly, however, the survey showed

Notes begin on p. 148. References begin on p. 155.

that only a fifth of the manuscripts had been revised before publication elsewhere, though the response rate to the questionnaire is too low for any firm conclusions to be drawn about these findings. A similar pattern emerged from another study, by Jean Wilson, the editor of a journal with a high impact factor, the *Journal of Clinical Investigation* (though he does not state the response rate to his questionnaire). In 1970 the *JCI* accepted 306 papers and rejected 149 (39). Again, 85 per cent of rejected articles were published elsewhere, in a 'distingished list of publications, with 14 journals accounting for one half of the papers,' and in only a sixth of cases were these changed before publication.

Hence for the *JCI* peer review had a significant impact on only a third of the rejected papers. Nevertheless, Wilson believes that the system is valid: further analysis showed that the citation rates for the articles published in the *JCI* were double those of the rejected articles published elsewhere.[1] Moreover, the authors of the 15 per cent of rejected articles that were not published, said that they had been convinced by peer review that their papers had been either unoriginal or wrong.

Garvey *et al.* confirmed this model in another discipline, psychology (16). Some 40 per cent of the articles had been rejected by the first journal to which they were submitted; two-thirds of them were submitted elsewhere and over 90 per cent were eventually published. Of 3676 published articles, 343 had been rejected by the first journal to which they had been submitted; half of the latter had not been revised before they were sent to another journal.

In assessing these findings one has to remember the difference between the acceptance rates of several 'core' journals and the others. Inevitably luck plays some part in getting a paper accepted in a journal with a high rejection rate and if authors regard acceptance as more of a lottery than related to quality they might be more likely to revise an article if it is rejected more than once. Anecdotally my British friends tell me that they will send an article to two general medical journals and a specialist one before thinking of revising it (then usually taking into account the referees' reports from the last journal). This practice was also found in the USA from a questionnaire sent to the authors of 172 papers accepted by the *American Journal of Public Health* between August 1983 and October 1984 (77). The *AJPH* has an acceptance rate of 20–45 per cent and, of the 172 accepted papers (the response rate to this questionnaire was 100 per cent), no fewer than 61 had been previously submitted to another journal. There had been 80 previous submissions to 25 different journals, half of them to the two American journals with the highest circulations, the *Journal of the American Medical Association* and the *New England Journal of Medicine.*

Almost a third of these 61 had been substantially revised before submission to the *AJPH* and a quarter moderately so; articles rejected by more than one journal were more likely to have been revised than those rejected only once. Irrespective of any previous revision, as a result of peer review by the *AJPH* 43 of the 61 articles were substantially revised or totally rewritten before they were published by the journal. Finally, a Medline search had shown that 40 per cent of the articles rejected by the *AJPH* had been published, eventually, though there are no data on whether these had been revised or not.

These findings were confirmed from the different viewpoint of an author's editor. Analysing 176 original articles coming through a regional medical editing centre, Mundy found that 30 per cent were accepted at the first attempt and 41 per cent at the second (78). The difference in acceptance rates probably arose because the author rewrote the article to take account of the referee's comments and because he chose the second journal more realistically. The total submission to publication time was 13·2 months and this was prolonged by only 2·5 months by the second, successful, attempt.

NEGATIVE EFFECTS

May editorial peer review still prevent good research from seeing the light of day? I know of no data for journal articles to answer this question, but there is some evidence of the influence of another type of peer review—that on research presented to meetings of scientific societies. In many of these, the abstracts are sent for peer review when they are submitted for presentation and a high proportion are rejected (currently 50 per cent for the British Society for Gastroenterology, for example). Nevertheless, even work that is presented often fails to be written up in full-length papers, and those that are published may show striking discrepancies between the original and the substantive work.

A Medline search showed that only 29 of the 51 abstracts of work presented at a meeting of the Surgical Research Society in 1972 had been published in full in the next three years (79). Possibly work presented at an early stage had been stillborn, the authors had not had the energy to complete it, or referees had condemned it. Similar results were found for cardiology from a computer search of 2765 randomly selected abstracts of presentations to the meetings of three societies (80). Half of these had led to full-length articles in peer reviewed journals within 37–43 months, but there was little difference between the citation rates of abstracts that had given rise to substantive articles and those that had not.

Why did half the abstracts fail to develop into substantive papers? No answer could be given, but it was concluded that citations of abstracts as references in articles should be discouraged. Nevertheless, apart from their brevity surely the quality of abstracts may be as good or as bad as that of full length articles (81). Many editors try to discourage their citation because they may mislead readers into thinking that they are definitive papers, but few journals have forbidden this.[2]

One journal that no longer allows the citation of abstracts has argued its case strongly (83). A study of seven consecutive spoken presentations at a paediatric specialty meeting in 1983 showed major discrepancies between these and the published abstracts, making the latter false. Even more disquietingly, at the 17th International Congress of

Paediatrics only two of the seven listed free presentations had been given—even though all seven were later printed in the published official proceedings.

Despite all this, it is important to emphasize that peer review for conference abstracts is not necessarily comparable with that for submitted papers: abstracts are usually reviewed fast, often 'blind', by a committee, and with a bias towards acceptance; substantive articles are usually reviewed deliberately, often non-blind, by one or two assessors, and with more of a likelihood of rejection initially than of acceptance.

MEASURES OF QUALITY

If, then, there is still much to learn about the fate of articles that journals reject, what can be said about the quality of the ones they publish? One answer comes from citation analysis: as we have seen, first rank scientists tend to publish papers that are highly cited in high impact factor journals (84), while highly cited papers are judged by consensus panels to be of higher quality than less cited papers (85).

One way of evaluating the individual published paper might be to look at the criticisms in the subsequent correspondence. But even remarkably bad articles may produce little or no comment; instead, poor work is often merely ignored. 'Negative' citations (articles which mention it only to criticize the findings) are rare and the failure of the article ever to appear as a reference is more frequent; in some disciplines, such as physics, between a quarter and a half of all papers are never cited (86).

Given that the results of citation analysis have some rough relationship with quality, how do citations correlate with the comments made by referees? For chemistry, Small studied a sample of 73 papers taken from the 4203 highly cited articles (more than 10 citations in one year) (87). Fifty of the authors provided usable replies about what the assessor had said: 23 sent the referees' reports, 12 could reconstruct them, and 15 said that their papers had been accepted without comment.

The recommendations in the reports were classified into four groups: publish unchanged; publish after minor revisions; publish after major revisions; and do not publish. These gradings were compared with the frequency of citations. The most highly cited papers had generally received the lowest evaluation by the assessors, and the distribution of the comments might have been expected by chance (though Small did not ask whether the articles had been revised before publication as a result of the referees' comments).

Small used another approach in assessing the quality of the articles: he asked a sample of chemists for their ratings. Again, these did not correlate with the referees' opinions. The major 'error of judgment' by a referee concerned the most highly cited article of all. This was now a standard reference, Small found, with 751 citations in eight years. In his report, however, the assessor had called for drastic revisions which unless made might lead to certain unjustified conclusions getting into the literature. The editor ignored these suggestions and published the article.

Small does not consider this misjudgment typical. Overall, for the middle of the road papers, peer review had worked efficiently and fairly, being controversial in only 10 per cent of instances. Given that the editor's judgment had been used, it had not prevented good work from being published (as in the most highly cited article). This is a good example of why the assessor's role must be as an adviser to the editor, and not the decision-maker, and the valuable part an editor may play in using his own judgment.

UNDETECTED ERRORS

A more direct way of assessing the adequacy of peer review is to look at the errors in published articles, particularly asking the main questions most editors pose: is the article original, scientifically reliable, and important for the discipline.

Originality is difficult to define. For example, does publication of a long abstract that includes data in the text, tables, or illustrations preclude publication of a formal article that contains no new results? Is a new paper in a 'salami' series of articles, which adds only a few cases to previous reports, substantial enough for acceptance (88)? Provided that they have been chosen correctly, however, at least reviewers should be able to identify work that has been published in a virtually identical form in another journal.

In their 'Instructions to Authors' most journals state that submission must be exclusive, and the 'Uniform Requirements for Manuscripts Submitted to Biomedical Journals' devotes a whole paragraph to prior and duplicate publication (82). Authors usually sign a copyright form stating that the articles are being submitted exclusively and have not been published elsewhere. Yet every editor can tell of examples where neither he nor the referee has detected that exactly or almost exactly the same work has already been published, without any mention of this by the author. Such duplication is particularly frequent between similar journals in Britain and Europe or the USA, between journals and books, or between journals and journal supplements devoted to conference proceedings. Some have called for action to deal with this, including a three-year ban on considering articles submitted by the offending authors (89). This seems to me too drastic and a better way is to publicize occurrences by printing a prominent notice about it in the journals concerned.

This failure by supposed experts to identify previously published work was highlighted by the study of Peter and Ceci: only three of the thirteen resubmitted papers were stated to be unoriginal (48). I suspect that this occurred because the referees were not chosen with enough care, or that they did not read the articles with enough attention. Nevertheless, another explanation is that these findings might be peculiar to psychology. For example, for at least four reasons they would be unlikely to be replicated in physics (19). Firstly, its subdisciplines are well delineated and active and spurious workers or research centres would have been recognized. Second, research in physics needs resources, so that there are a limited number of institutions where the research could have been carried out. Third, research in physics is cumulative; a research topic that was three years out of date should have been closed and the resubmitted papers would have aroused suspicions. Finally, there is the grapevine, so that the invisible colleges would have known about the work already before it was published.

Another discipline which an editor commenting on the Peters and Ceci article thought would have detected the resubmission is statistics (90). The *Journal of the American Statistical Association* uses a preliminary screen of 10–15 associate editors, with a full review by two referees if the paper seems plausible.

Nevertheless, although the editors might not have been expected to recognize the articles (91), this should have been a requirement for the referees. So were they suffering from information overload—a question that Waksman has asked in a different context (32)? With the flood of new articles and the increased rejection and resubmission rates, many new and inexperienced referees were now being used, with a resultant decline in the quality of assessment. If Waksman is right, it also reflects a decline in editoral standards, for one of the editor's main tasks is to monitor his advisers. He should choose the right ones for a particular paper, help them over assessing it, and not continue to use them if they consistently produce inadequate opinions.

REASON FOR NON-RECOGNITION

The idea of incompetence was supported by an experienced observer of peer review, John Ziman (92), who had never come across standards as low as those shown in the study by Peters and Ceci; were the reviewers sufficiently well qualified? So do we accept the charge or are there valid reasons why the articles should not have been recognized as unoriginal?

One of the failings of editors is that they believe people read everything published in their journals. Yet the readership of an individual article may be remarkably small. Another historian of science, De Solla Price, has shown how a journal's circulation is often equivalent to the subscriptions of the authors who are publishing in it, together with sales to libraries; the 'authorship' makes up the journal's regular readership (possibly as small as 200–300) (15). And such an authorship may not be a high proportion of the workers in that discipline: of 10,000 psychologists, probably only 1000 were active in research, producing an article every two or three years (16).

Given that the predominant work in science is 'mop-up' rather than innovative (93); that the papers studied by Peters and Ceci were probably not very important (the mean annual citation figure was said to have been low (1·9) and in any case there may have been self-citations (94)); and that only 0·5–1·0 per cent of psychologists read any article, perhaps the failure of the assessors to recognize the articles might have been predicted (95). Thus if an article has a 9 in 10 chance of not being read by a general reader, including the editor and his adviser, then the probability that two reviewers and one editor will not recognize it is $(0·9)^3$—that is, 0·73.

Another reason for not recognizing an article that has already been published is that many scientists do not read the journals produced in other countries, even the major ones. British workers often say that it is a feature of American scientists to ignore British publications, and the French complain that the Anglo-Saxons fail to cite their work (96). I have no data but I am struck by how frequently American review articles on, say, a new anti-asthma agent or beta-blocker fail to mention the original publications on the drug in the *BMJ* or a British or Scandinavian specialty journal.

An additional factor in the Peters and Ceci case is the lag of a year between submission and publication. Added to the delay of 18–32 months before they resubmitted the published work, the effective age of the research was $2\frac{1}{2}$–$3\frac{1}{2}$ years. In this period a referee in his role as a scientist would probably read 1000 articles; he may remember the general aspects of the article, but not its provenance, and hence fall back on dismissing it because of 'methodological flaws' rather than wasting time determining where it had been published (95). Such flaws may have been obvious to the original reviewers, who nevertheless recommended that the articles should be accepted.

Some commentators mentioned that a whisper of plagiarism in an assessor's report is a serious accusation—which might hazard a junior referee's career—and blander comments about flaws in methods and interpretation would be just as effective in advising the editor to reject the article (97). Yet, like piracy and fraud, plagiarism has recently hit the headlines and illustrated another pitfall for peer review.

PLAGIARISM

Further evidence of delays in the recognition of published work has come from recent reports of piracy and plagiarism, other abuses that editors and reviewers have to be on the look out for. In the late 1970s Elias A. K. Alsabti, an Iraqi working at various centres in the USA, published some 60 papers, most if not all pirated or plagiarized from other people's work. He retyped a published paper, removed the author's name and substituted his own, and then submitted it to an obscure journal (98). Two-thirds of a review article printed under Alsabti's name was published in identical forms in two European cancer journals and was an almost verbatim copy of part of one of his professor's grant applications, to which he had access while working in the laboratory (99).

Among other journals, Alsabti's papers were published in the *Journal of Cancer Research and Clinical Oncology, Japanese Journal of Experimental Medicine, Journal of Clinical Haematology and Oncology*, and *British Journal of Urology*. Though the text was usually identical, the title might be changed. For example, one article that Alsabti pirated was entitled 'Suppression of spleen lymphocyte mitogenesis in mice injected by platinum compounds'. Sent to a reviewer at the MD Anderson Hospital who had been dead for two years, it was picked up by Alsabti, who made a few changes, added his own name and that of two fictitious authors, and altered the title to 'Effect of platinum compounds on murine lymphocyte mitogenesis'. This was published in the *Japanese Journal of Medical Science and Biology* before the original was printed in the *European Journal of Cancer*.

Discussing Alsabti's career in their book *Betrayers of the Truth*, Broad and Wade cite at least four other plagiarists who built up considerable bibliographies of works written by others which were not detected by the ordinary editorial processes but emerged under various circumstances (100) and doubtless there are many others. A common feature was that, although the work was trivial, it was eventually published, often in an obscure journal, and failed to be cited.

STATISTICAL FAULTS

Do reviewers also fail to detect major errors in articles written in good faith? They cannot be expected, of course, always to recognize work that is flawed, for more research may be needed to show this. Yet at least they should be able to spot errors in the statistical aspect of a study—not necessarily mathematical errors (though these occur) but more the faulty logic of the data collection, analysis, and interpretation. As a result of these findings many of us have introduced a separate check by an expert statistician after the article has been provisionally approved for publication.

An early example of a survey of statistics in medical articles was published in 1966 (101). Schor and Karten chose 10 of the most frequently read American medical journals and asked experienced biostatisticians to read 25 articles in each (usually in three issues published in 1964). Were the conclusions valid for the design of the experiment, what about the type of analysis, and were the statistical tests applicable?

Schor and Karten found twelve types of error occurring in the analytical articles.[3] Nevertheless, such deficiencies made less than 28 per cent of the papers unacceptable for publication even if no changes were to have been made, and only 5 per cent were unsalvageable.

A similar study of 62 articles published in the *BMJ* in 1976 showed at least one error in 32 of these (14 of commission—abuse of statistics—10 of omission, and 8 of both). Five of the articles made claims in their abstracts that were not supported by the data presented (102). The reason given for such low standards was that no statistician had been concerned either in the design of the study or as an assessor in evaluating the paper for publication (103). In consequence, subjects and resources had been wasted, standards of treatment had been poor, other research might have been affected, and subsequent studies might have used the same substandard methods. Criticism in the correspondence columns could not be guaranteed and hence was not an adequate safeguard.

Comparable findings have been presented for reports of clinical trials in four main general medical journals; again, there was a frequent failure to mention eligibility criteria, method of randomization, blind assessment, and power of the study (104).

All these studies have had a powerful effect, if only by heightening awareness of poor planning and analysis. If one of the major preoccupations of medical editors in the 1960s and 1970s has been with ethics, in the 1980s and 1990s it is likely to be with statistics. Such findings have, however, to be put into perspective even if the views sound old fashioned. Firstly, clinical importance should not be confused with statistical significance. Nor must it be forgotten that there is still great scope for simple observational studies, as shown recently with the early reports on the acquired immune deficiency syndrome (AIDS). There is a danger that authors may be put off writing such reports if there is an over-emphasis on statistical niceties. Finally, statistics are much more subjective than most of us realize and there are legitimate differences among experts over many aspects. That said, however, having used expert statistical evaluation for five years, I would not return to peer review without it; it now has a major role for us and many of our specialty journals.

THERAPEUTIC TRIALS

Similar studies have been done on deficiencies in articles which peer review has failed to detect. Thus a checklist was used to analyze the soundness of all reports of therapeutic trials published in four British medical journals (two weekly and two monthly) between 1 January and 1 June 1966 and 1969 (105). Of 141 trials, 51 per cent were definitely acceptable, 16 per cent were probably acceptable, and 33 per cent unacceptable. Most of the articles in the first two categories had been published in the weekly journals. The unacceptable papers were characterized by inadequate or inappropriate methods, absent or inadequate controls, and unreported statistics.

A survey some years later, however, showed that the recommendations made in the light of these findings had not been applied to a similar problem—the reporting of drug side effects. In only 55 per cent of 5737 articles was sufficient information given to enable the rate of an adverse drug reaction to be calculated (106). A comparison of articles published in 1972–3, when some recommendations had been made, and 1975–9 showed that no significant change had occurred. Such surveys, I believe, have done a large amount of good: they have given rise to checklists which can be used by authors, assessors, and editors, freeing the latter two at least to concentrate on other aspects of the article.

FRAUD

One of the most publicized limitations of peer review has been the revelation of several serious instances of fraud—data that had been invented and incorporated in articles that were subsequently accepted for publication. The most notorious case, perhaps is that of Sir Cyril Burt, who for years hoodwinked scientists and the public about the alleged connections between inheritance and intelligence. In medicine he has a counterpart in John Darsee, who during cardiovascular research posts at both Emory University and

51

Harvard published 45 articles, of which 44 are invalid. Most of the data were invented, his co-authors were sometimes not told of the work being published, and in several papers the co-authors were apparently fictitious (107).

In some ways Darsee's story is a modern morality tale, in which few emerge with much merit, throwing light on our standards and ambitions. In 1981 he was detected falsifying data and his NIH fellowship was stopped by his chief, who, concluding that the incident was an isolated one, told the Dean of Harvard Medical School but not the National Heart, Lung, and Blood Institute. Later it became clear that Darsee's data for a collaborative study did not tally with those produced at three other centres. Subsequent investigations showed that he had systematically falsified data in at least five animal research studies at Harvard and in many earlier studies in a previous post at Emory University. Most of the articles and abstracts were retracted by their co-authors in the journals that had published them.

Although we might echo that there is 'no spectacle so ridiculous as the [British] public in one of its periodical fits of morality', this story of Darsee's falsifications, two commentators suggested, shows flaws in the supervision of research in academic centres, lax attitudes over the authorship of articles, and weakness in peer review for journals and books (107). To be fair, however, it needed time for the very idea of fraud to sink into people's consciousness; even now, most of us assume that scientists are honest, and that, though data may be wrong, they are not invented. The next five or ten years will show whether now that reviewers recognize the possibility of fraud and there is a code for dealing with newly discovered instances it will diminish. But we know that this major episode was not an isolated instance: another major university, Yale, was implicated in fraud in an episode which was directly connected with peer review (108). This arose when a junior colleague of a head of department, when sent an article on glucose metabolism in anorexia nervosa to review, advised its rejection by the *New England Journal of Medicine*, and then prepared a similar paper with invented data and several items purloined from the original manuscript. After the subsequent inquiry 11 previous papers had to be retracted, in nine cases because the data had disappeared; in seven of these papers the department head had been a co-author.

In the next few months other instances of forged data came to light: in 1983 alone there were reports of four major instances. Joseph Cort had fabricated data in two scientific papers, a patent application, and a National Institutes of Health grant application for research into two vasopressin analogues and two LHRH antagonists, none of which had been synthesized (the work being published in the *International Journal of Peptide Research* and *Advances in the Physiological Sciences* (109)). William S. Aronow, a Long Beach cardiologist, confessed to irregularities in various studies, an NIH inquiry having found discrepancies in five studies on four different drugs, all favouring their efficacy (including prazosin and timolol in angina) (110). Karl Illmensee, professor of embryology at Geneva, lost an NIH grant, with the investigating committee being unable to decide whether there had been an 'element of invention' in his mammalian nuclear manipulation experiments in mice (111). Michael Purves resigned his readership in physiology at Bristol University, having acknowledged that his data on 5 deoxyglucose metabolism by the sheep fetal brain during sleep given to the 28th International Physiology Congress were false (112).

In *Betrayers of the Truth* Broad and Wade record these and many other earlier instances of scientific fraud, some speculative and others definite (100). They point out that peer review had not detected these; for example, Long had published photographs of chromosomes alleged to be human but which were not.

Angell, a deputy editor of the *New England Journal of Medicine*, has emphasized the editor's role in preventing the publication of fraudulent work by getting work vetted by experts (113). The latter would often spot deficiencies in methods or inconsistencies in the results and might know of questions about the integrity of earlier work by the same researchers. Editors should feel free to ask for more data, and to reject the article if the response was unsatisfactory.

With all this talk of fraud it might be asked whether we are back to the days of Robert Boyle's 'philosophicall robbery', which publication in a peer reviewed journal was supposed to stop. We cannot answer for certain, though if fraud were common surely more cases should have been reported. We have few data, particularly about those false results which are detected by referees and are therefore not published (anecdotally, for instance, I have heard several accounts from professors about pirated theses, copied out by a PhD candidate from dusty originals in a library. The penalty is expulsion from the university, but publicity is rare). Even for published work at least one major journal has so far refused to publish retractions of fraudulent work, maintaining that it is the *JCI* not the FBI (114). (Most of us, however, have misinterpreted Majerus's remark: Dr Thomas Stossel tells me that what he actually meant was that the *JCI* did not have the FBI's resources to do the necessary rigorous investigation.)

Even if major forgery is rare, however, lesser misdemeanours may be more common. Authors may omit data that do not support their thesis or smooth off curves to give the required result; a helpful referee may find that his comments have been transformed into somebody else's publication; or a referee may photostat an article sent for review and use it in his own work.

Such purloining of ideas may be common. No fewer than a fifth of 300 cancer research workers who had been denied grants by the NIH stated that their data had been pirated by reviewers (100). Finally some sharp practices that a few know about may not be published: in the discussion of the cardiological studies by William Aronow, who undertook not to carry out research in the future, it emerged that seven similar undertakings had been given and that 50 researchers had been officially disqualified (113). Nevertheless, editors of journals had not been told about all this, and, given that Aronow's studies had been prominent in establishing standards for carbon monoxide in ambient air, Rapaport, the editor of *Circulation*, was indignant that they had not been informed.

ERRORS IN REFEREE'S REPORT

How common are errors in the referee's report itself? We try to pick these out, on the basis of our own knowledge or of that of members of the hanging committee or of the author's riposte to the referees' reports; another source are points made in subsequent 'Letters to the Editor'.

Most authors resent adverse comments, particularly if they have been the basis for the article's rejection, but there has been little systematic study of their accuracy. Nevertheless, Horrobin, a fervent critic of peer review (particularly for research grants), has estimated that a third of assesors' reports are accurate, competent, and fair; another third are accurate but obsessed with the trivial; and a third are inaccurate on objective grounds (115). Waksman also commented that today referees wasted their time making capricious or inept criticism; in any issue of the *Journal of Immunology* it was not unusual to see half a dozen papers in which the principal references had not been cited (32), to which presumably the referees had not drawn attention.

Not uncommonly authors also complain about the acerbic and derisive flavour of many reports, Ingelfinger detailing some of the words they use: 'naive, ridiculous, gross stupidity, waste of effort and money, lacking all qualification' (116). Any such judgments should be supported by documentary evidence, as should other general statements (117). Yet another of the editor's tasks is to censor such wounding comments out of any report which is to be sent to an author. Many editors ask for personal comments to be made in a separate letter, yet some referees seem to have a hidden cruel streak which they cannot resist using. In the *BMJ* office we use a lot of Tippex (an eraser) on these reports, but occasionally we miss a wounding statement. I know of one referee's report (not for the *BMJ*) which, sent uncensored and not in an envelope marked 'Personal', almost provoked a libel action (and I suspect that this might have been successful).

5

Research: a personal survey

Research (1694). *Investigation, inquiry into things.*

I suppose it was the spectacle of Clegg and Fox, both powerful editors producing good journals in different ways, that set me thinking whether it could be shown that editorial peer review was effective. So in 1979 I set up a prospective study into its process and outcome as used by the *BMJ*. This aimed at determining the contribution made at each of the different stages of peer review, as well as the fate of the articles that were rejected. In particular, was consensus between readers (whether expert referees or not) better than by chance and did peer review by experts produce better results than those by an editor alone? My study was designed to examine these questions, keeping conditions as normal as possible.

Nowadays the *Lancet* relies heavily on peer review, 90 per cent of its published articles having been evaluated by outside experts (Munro, personal communication). Under its previous editors, however, most assessments were made in house, the practice being defended by its last editor. Ian Douglas-Wilson (25). Peer review, he thought, was slow, conservative and élitist, and possibly bigoted. Without it mistakes might be no more frequent than with it—though admittedly they might be more massive; though the risks were relatively great, so were the rewards, particularly in the speed of publication.

Coming from the editor of a leading medical journal, Douglas-Wilson's statements command respect, but, like many other pronouncements on this subject, they were unsupported by rigorous analysis. Despite his opinion (discussed more fully on p. 91) and all the views and fragmentary evidence against peer review, why has the system persisted for over 300 years, and become almost

Notes begin on p. 148. References begin on p. 157.

universal? Is there any evidence of its value, should we try to improve both the process and the outcome (and if so, how), does peer review for research grants have the same problems, and what light do any findings that we have throw on science itself and the people who work in it? These are the themes of my remaining chapters.

STUDY: MATERIALS AND METHODS

The study was prospective, computer-based, and covered every consecutive article submitted to the *BMJ* between 1 January and 15 August 1979. After a pilot study of 50 articles I devised a form giving essential details of each article, including its subject matter, total length of individual sections, and number of tables, illustrations, and authors.

Four groups of readers were used in assessing the articles: the editor (SPL), a colleague (DS), an expert referee, and the hanging committee. Each reader made an individual assessment of the articles on a four-point scale (poor, moderate, considerable, high). They scored four criteria: originality, scientific reliability, clinical importance, suitability for publication in the *BMJ*. Finally, each of them gave a recommendation: accept for publication in the *BMJ*; accept for publication after modification; unsuitable for *BMJ*; unsuitable for publication in any journal.

Each reader completed the form about the article without reference to the judgments of others. He also scored each criterion (such as originality) independently of the other criteria. SPL scored the overall opinion of the hanging committee on the articles it discussed. The remaining details on the form were filled in by SPL. He was also present at the hanging committee to record judgments, but took no part in the discussions.

Outcome

The outcome was assessed as follows. If the paper was published by *BMJ*, SPL filled in the following details on the form:

Was the article changed?	Yes/No
If changed, which aspect?	Shortening/scientific style
If changed, by whom?	Author/editor/both
If changed, how much?	0–25/21–50/51–75/76+%

If the article was rejected by *BMJ*, a year later the author was sent a questionnaire containing the following queries:

Was the article published elsewhere?	Yes/No
If published elsewhere	Where?
If published elsewhere was it altered?	Yes/No

The questionnaire to the author was repeated twice if necessary. Authors who did not reply were asked about the fate of their articles by a personal letter or telephone call, or this was ascertained from the *Index Medicus* for the next three years, or, finally, from a Medline search.

The impact factor of the journals in which rejected articles were published was obtained from the 1979 *Science Citation Index*. The impact factors were then grouped by numbers and an arbitrary scale constructed. This ranged from 0 to 8 and on it the *BMJ* ranked 6. Impact factors in groups 6 to 8 were classified as high.

The assessment of results was in three main ways. Firstly, whether the article was published at all. Second, according to the impact factor of the journal—a 'good' outcome being publication in a journal with a high impact factor (including the *BMJ*). Third, the level of consensus between the readers was determined, the higher the agreement above chance the better.

Finally, as a check on the use of the impact factor as a criterion, the citations to a small but statistically valid random sample of 39 papers accepted by the *BMJ* were compared with those of 39 articles rejected by the *BMJ* and published elsewhere and those of 39 articles that had reached the hanging committee stage but had still been rejected and published elsewhere.

All the data were transferred to a computer for analysis of both longitudinal and correlative trends. Statistical evaluation was performed by χ^2 and kappa tests for agreement between readers (118).

STUDY: RESULTS, AND COMMENT

A total of 1558 articles was received. Of these, seven were unavailable for analysis (six had been wrongly coded and put into the scheme and in one documentation was lost).

Types of article
Of the 1551 articles remaining for analysis, 997 had been submitted as Original Articles, 492 as Short Reports, 33 as Medical Practice contributions, 18 as (scientific) Letters to the Editor, 4 as For Debate articles, and 7 others. A 'typical' original article was 1500 words long, and had three authors, one illustration, two tables and 13 references.

The flow chart of the 1551 manuscripts and their fate is shown in figure 4. From the questionnaire, *Index Medicus*, and Medline the outcome for 1143 of the 1223 rejected articles (93 per cent) is known: 836 (68 per cent) were published elsewhere and 307 (25 per cent) were not published; the outcome is unknown for 80 papers (7 per cent).

Fate of articles
Of the 1551 articles, 825 were rejected in the office after appraisal by two medically qualified readers and 726 were sent to an external specialist referee. Of the latter, 489 were sent to the editorial committee and 328 were accepted for publication. Thus the acceptance rate was 328/1551= 21 per cent.

Rejected articles
Of the total of 1143 rejected papers with a known outcome, 836 were published elsewhere, 130 (16 per cent) of them in journals with high impact factors. Only 20 per cent of these articles were changed before being published.

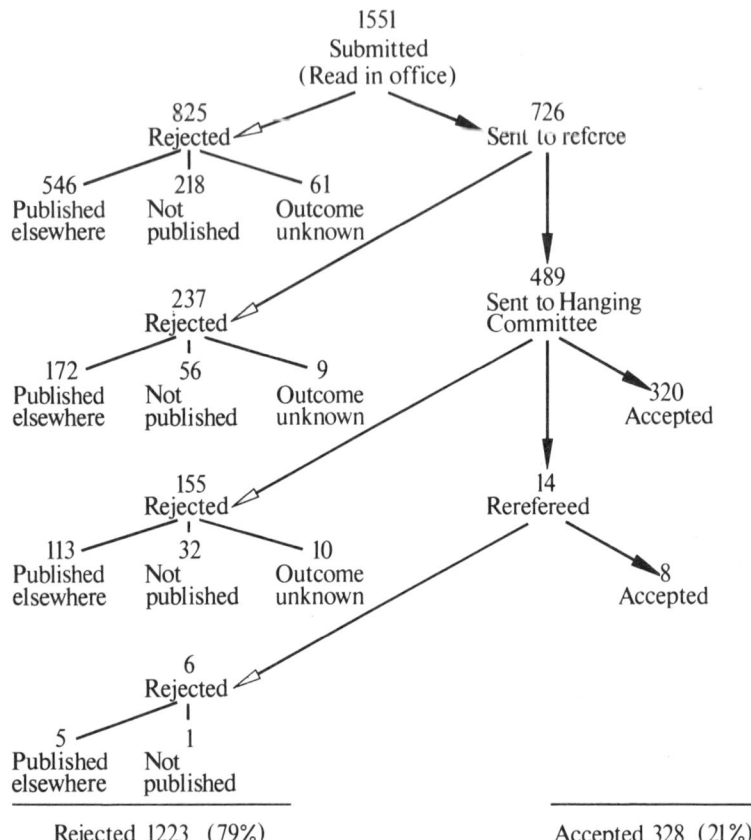

FIGURE 4. Fate of 1551 consecutive articles submitted for publication to the *BMJ* in 1979.

There was no significant difference in the proportion of all types of papers accepted by the *BMJ*, except for Short Reports (13 per cent accepted, compared with 25 per cent for Original Articles; $\chi^2=27\cdot4$, df$=3$, p$<0\cdot001$).

Authors
Slightly over half of all the articles submitted were written by authors holding an academic appointment and these were

Table VIII. Acceptance of papers and qualification of author.

Authors	No submitted	No (%) accepted
Only medical	1076	201 (19)
No medical	51	5 (10)
Both medical and non-medical	424	122 (29)
	1551	328

$$(\chi^2=22\cdot6; \ df = 2; \ p<0\cdot001)$$

significantly more likely to have their papers accepted than non-academic ones (24 per cent accepted versus 18 per cent; $\chi^2=9\cdot1$; $df=1$; $p<0\cdot001$). Most papers (1076) had only medical authors, but a few (51) had none; the 424 articles with both medical and non-medical authors had a significantly greater chance of being accepted than the other two categories (table VIII).

Referees
Of the total of 246 referees used, 143 held academic appointments and 103 service posts. Although papers with academic authors were more likely to be sent to a referee than those with no academic authors, and were more likely to be sent to an academic rather than a service referee, this did not effect the outcome. The proportions of papers accepted (with either academic or service authors) did not differ according to the type of referee. There was no evidence of status bias, academic referees judging papers by academic or non-academic authors to an equal standard, and vice versa (table IX).

Outcome
The outcome was good for 130 of the 1223 articles rejected by the *BMJ*—these being published in journals with an impact factor equal to or higher than that of the *BMJ*; 83 of these were in general journals (table X). The proportion of papers published in general journals with high impact factors that were rejected after being read by the referees or

Table IX. Flow of papers and author and referee status.

	No of papers received	No sent to referee	No accepted	No sent to acad. ref.	No sent to service ref.	No accepted by: Acad. ref.	Serv. ref.
Academic authors:	858 (55%)	451 (53%)	206 (24%)	319 (71%)	132 (29%)	142 (45%)	64 (49%)
Non-academic authors:	693 (45%)	275 (40%)	122 (18%)	154 (56%)	121 (44%)	68 (44%)	54 (45%)
	1551 (100%)	726	328	473	253	210	118

Table X. Rejected papers published in high impact factor journals.

	Total rejected	Total published elsewhere	No published in journals with high IFs 6–8	No (%) in general journals with high IFs
Rejected in office	825	546	76	40 (5%) (Lancet 30, BMJ 6*)
Rejected by referee	237	172	30	24 (10%) (Lancet 20, BMJ 4*)
Rejected by 'hanging committee'	161	118	24	19 (12%) (Lancet 15, BMJ 4*)
Total	1223	836	130	83 (70%)

* Some articles were resubmitted to the BMJ after the study and ultimately accepted.

hanging committee was significantly greater than the proportion rejected after being read by the office editor. The analysis of actual citations of three groups of papers (table XI) showed that those papers published in the BMJ had a significantly higher citation rate than either of the two groups of rejected papers. Those rejected by the hanging committee also had a higher citation rate than those rejected at any stage.

Of the 328 articles accepted by the BMJ, 270 (82 per cent) were revised. Over half of these (169) were changed 'scientifically'—for example, further data were added or additional details of the methods or statistical analysis given. Almost half had alterations in style, usually shortening (done by the technical editor in two-thirds of the cases).

Recommendations

For the 1551 papers, the referees successfully recommended a significantly higher proportion of acceptances by the BMJ than either SPL or one of his colleagues (table XII).

Table XI. Citations for three groups of papers up to 1984.

	Accepted by *BMJ* (n=39)	Rejected by *BMJ*	
		Rejected by hanging committee (n=39)	Rejected at any stage (n=39)
Citations per year	1·82	1·64	0·9
	($\chi^2=66\cdot5$; df=2; p<0·001)		

Table XII. Proportion of papers recommended for acceptance or rejection by individual editors or referees that were actually accepted by BMJ.

	Proportion recommended for acceptance that were accepted	Proportion recommended for rejection that were accepted
	1551 papers	
SPL	0·74	0·08
DS	0·43	0·04
Referee*	0·74	0·10
	489 papers	
SPL	0·84	0·45
DS	0·71	0·44
Referee†	0·74	0·35

* These include both external referees and internal ones (those office colleagues who gave a second opinion when the original editor thought the paper should be rejected).
† These are entirely external referees.

CONSENSUS

Overall

In all cases consensus between various judges was higher than by chance—and in all cases it was higher for the 1551 articles than it was for the 489 that went to the hanging committee (table XIII).

Table XIII. *Agreement on recommendations on 1551 and 489 articles (%).*

	Actual agreement (%)	Chance agreement (%)	K	P value
		1551		
SPL/DS	70	53	0·36	<0·001
SPL/REF*	81	63	0·49	<0·001
REF*/DS	74	53	0·45	<0·001
		489		
SPL/DS	59	54	0·11	<0·01
SPL/HC	72	52	0·42	<0·001
HC/DS	69	63	0·17	<0·001
HC/REF†	73	62	0·31	<0·001

* Referee here includes both internal and external referees.
† External referees only.

Referee v SPL

A separate analysis was performed on the subset of 707[1] articles seen by the external reviewer. His judgments on the four criteria and recommendations were compared with those of SPL to see whether each criterion related to the recommendation.

The levels of agreement for the individual judgments were: originality 62 per cent (chance 52 per cent); scientific reliability 64 per cent (chance 54 per cent); clinical importance 68 per cent (chance 52 per cent); suitability 64 per cent (chance 54 per cent). These figures are similar to the overall level of agreement on the final recommendation on acceptance or rejection (65 per cent compared with 49 per cent expected by chance ($P < 0·001$)), and all were significantly better than chance.

Each judgment on an individual criterion was related to the recommendation in a positive way, most strongly for suitability and clinical importance for SPL and suitability for the referee.

Hanging committee v the rest

Analysis of the subset of 489 articles that went to the hanging committee showed a level of agreement higher than by chance (table XIII). SPL agreed most with the hanging committee on importance, while the office editor and the referee agreed with it most on originality.

DISCUSSION

As several others have found (2,7,39), studies on peer review are difficult, partly because the process is difficult to measure, and partly because we lack a 'gold standard' for outcome. Nevertheless, my study did produce four important results. The *BMJ* 'captured' four-fifths of the articles that were published in high impact factor general journals; consensus between readers was better, often much better, than by chance; as a result of the assessors' recommendations most of the articles we published were substantially changed; and the whole 'system', using editors, referee, and hanging committee, seemed to work—that is, each stage seemed to filter out the less acceptable papers, leaving better and better subsets.

I will now consider the difficulties of the study and their findings in turn.

Methods

Different reviewers have different backgrounds and experience of peer review, their judgments on criteria such as originality and scientific reliability vary considerably, and their final recommendations about acceptance or rejection may be associated with different values for the different criteria. One referee may score all criteria as moderate and recommend acceptance; another may score all as considerable and recommend rejection to a specialist journal. (This phenomenon has been observed by other editors and is known to anthropologists as intersubjectivity (117)). In my study, for example, DS consistently judged well over

66

half the papers as moderate in each category but considered that more were acceptable than did other readers.

These difficulties might have been diminished by specifying the criteria for acceptance of an article. I rejected this, however, because I wanted to mimic real life as far as possible ('Wie es eigentlich gewesen ist' (As things really were), as Ranke said should be the aim of the historian (119)). Acceptance of an article is the responsibility of the editor, aided by his hanging committee, and not of the referee (though he is asked for a recommendation). Another problem was that the use of gradings and a form was already a departure from *BMJ* practice, and a few referees did not like them.

Measurement of outcome

Our overall acceptance rate was 21 per cent, roughly the same as that of several other major general journals. Some 68 per cent of the rejected articles were published elsewhere, 15 per cent in high impact factor journals, and 10 per cent in high impact factor general journals, again similar to the experience of others (39,47). The problem is to say whether we accepted the 'right' articles or not and to define some sort of 'gold standard' for doing this.

Like that of Jean Wilson, the editor of the *Journal of Clinical Investigation,* my gold standard was based on citation analysis, comparing the impact factors of the journals publishing the articles we had rejected with the impact factor of the *BMJ* (39). Wilson found that articles accepted by the *JCI* had double the average number of citations of those rejected and published elsewhere.

I used a different method for evaluating the quality of the articles—the impact factor of the journal publishing these. There were both logistical and scientific reasons for this. Firstly, the delay after publication required for a rigorous citation analysis would have doubled the length of the study. Second, the cost and the work entailed would have been beyond our resources. Third, there is evidence that the impact factor of a journal is as valid a measurement of quality as the citation rates of the individual articles. It may even eliminate some of the (admittedly only occasional) inconsistencies such as personal citations, or negative citations (120). Given that the whole topic of citation analysis is controversial, I believe that this method was valid, a view which is supported by the statistically significant differences in the small-scale study of citations of the three groups of articles.

The analysis of outcome suggested that the whole system of using editors and referees to filter out unacceptable and unsuitable papers, leaving the hanging committee to choose from among a group of potentially acceptable papers, was working efficiently. Firstly, papers accepted by the *BMJ* had higher average citations than those it rejected; and those rejected by the hanging committee had higher average citations than those rejected at any stage. Second, the fact that a higher proportion of papers rejected by the hanging committee and referee than by the office editors ended up in high impact factor journals also suggested that the referee and, particularly, the hanging committee were dealing with higher quality papers. The loss of 83 papers (5 per cent) to general journals with high impact factors did not seem too disturbing out of a total cohort of 1551.

Recommendations

For the 1551 papers, the referees successfully recommended a significantly higher proportion of acceptances by the *BMJ* than did either SPL or one of his colleagues (table XII). Obviously the hanging committee (which took the decision) was likely to have been strongly influenced by the referee, so it cannot be inferred that the referee was 'capturing' significantly more articles than the other participants, but at least there was no evidence that he had a negative influence.

Consensus

In all cases consensus was higher for the 1551 articles than it was for the 489 that went to the hanging committee (tables VI and VII). Almost certainly this is because (as others have found (2)) there was more agreement on which were the 'bad' articles in the larger group than in the smaller group.

Consensus was better than that expected by chance, being roughly of the same order as that found for other medical journals—that is, between 64 and 81 per cent, compared with 52–63 per cent expected by chance. Consensus between the various groups was roughly the same for all the categories and tallied more or less with the final recommendation.

There has been much discussion about the low consensus between two or more assessors about a single article, some commentators implying that because it was not all that much higher than by chance peer review was not valid for judging articles, and that low consensus applied particularly to medical articles.

Nevertheless, I believe that too much emphasis has been placed on consensus. After all, Peters and Ceci showed high levels of this, but the editors and referees had failed to detect unoriginal work, commenting instead on the poor scientific rigour of articles that had already been published and achieved modest citation rates. And there is the cogent view that referees should be deliberately chosen for opposite attributes and that when two agree completely from the outset one of them may be redundant (120).

Changes in articles

A major role for referees is, I believe, in helping to refine the article. Over half of the articles published in the *BMJ* were changed as a result of their suggestions, compared with only 20 per cent of the articles which we rejected and were published elsewhere. Similar results have been reported: revision for only 20 per cent for papers rejected by the *New England Journal of Medicine*, or for 15 per cent for those rejected by the *Journal of Clinical Investigation* (39,47). (This aspect is discussed on p. 40).

CONCLUSIONS

Though designed to analyze the role of the three stages in editorial evaluation of original articles for the *BMJ* (office editor, referee, and hanging committee), as well as the fate of the articles the journal rejected, this study did not answer the first question fully—in particular, whether the *BMJ* could have done without the expert referee. It did show, however, that 68 per cent of the articles the *BMJ* rejected were published elsewhere, most (but not all) in specialist journals with lower impact factors and most of them unchanged. Moreover, an appreciable proportion of articles (25 per cent) remained unpublished, possibly because their authors were convinced by peer review that they were wrong. The authors of four-fifths of the unpublished articles replied to my questionnaire, so that at least I know for certain that they did not resubmit the articles.

MAJOR DIFFICULTIES

Patterson and Bailar have commented on the paradox that editors, the arbiters of rigour, quality, and innovativeness in publishing scientific work, do not apply to their own work the standards they apply to judging the work of others (35). In mounting any such study, there are two major categories of difficulties (which they acknowledge in a subsequent article (121)).

The first category is in studying the process, which has at least four individual components.

Mechanical aspects
These comprise documenting the flow of papers through the journal (and also to other journals if the articles are rejected). If blinding (of the referee, or editor, or preferably both) is to be a feature of the study, then the logistical problems will be increased considerably.

Help for the reviewer
The reviewer needs more help, such as guidelines and

checklists, and any study should ensure consistency of definitions among members of the advisory team.

Advice taken

The editor must ensure that referees note any advice (for, like authors who fail to follow 'Instruction to Authors' and book reviewers who ignore guidelines, I suspect that many referees would ignore any guidelines, preferring to go on as they had always done).

Factors in the process

All the factors in the process that need to be studied must be included. According to Patterson and Bailar, these include: the quality of the published paper; where a paper is published; inter-referee agreement (and, if absent, the reason); the editor's influence on fairness; and the costs of the reviewing system. I would add at least one more: finding out from the authors if the paper had already been rejected by another journal before it came to the journal undertaking the study.

Given that Patterson and Bailar also suggest that the study sample should be clearly defined and that a random sample of journals should be used (to evaluate any influence of the discipline), such a research programme will clearly not be for the fainthearted (or the part-timer).

The second category of difficulty is in devising a gold standard. Should this be citation rates, journal impact factor, or inclusion as a standard reference into the body of knowledge, such as textbooks or review articles at, say, ten or more years after publication? Any of these has its virtues, but any may also be faulted, even the last—as in the case of Krebs cycle. In the 20 years 1962–81 this was cited explicitly only about 30 times—an example of the 'obliteration phenomenon', which occurs when something has become common wisdom in a discipline (122).

This is not to say, of course, that editors should not be trying to improve peer review, by improving the process and trying to measure the outcome. I will make some suggestions for both of these later in this book.

6

Parallels: peer review, science, and medicine

Parallel (1604). Having the same or a like course, tendency, or purport.

Totally unfettered research or publication would achieve little. If all scientists were entitled to a research grant, then the individual sums would be small and inevitably the difficult researchers would argue that their projects deserved more. If some were to be allowed larger grants than others, then a choice would have to be made with some sort of review process. Given that most research is now funded by the state, the ordinary citizen/taxpayer would call for a fair method of evaluation. As we have found with the Health Service (123), publicly funded organizations costing millions of pounds a year cannot escape external scrutiny; the priority is to ensure that this is fair and disinterested.

The same is true of publication. For a journal to print everything submitted to it might lead to chaos, as well as bankruptcy. True, perhaps not too much long-term scientific harm might be done. After ten years the bad articles would have clumped together in a sediment, ignored and uncited ever since they were published. Some of the good papers might have been recognized, refined and added to by further work, and incorporated into the knowledge base of the subject. In the meantime, however, readers might have been confused, particularly by claims made outside their own disciplines, while good work might have been obscured by the bad.

Such an experiment in uncontrolled scientific publishing has recently been proposed (124), but it has already been tried (125). For five years, from 1961 the National Institutes of Health experimented with rapid dissemination of unevaluated preprints. Participants in these 'information exchange groups' sent their manuscripts to the NIH, which copied and forwarded them to other members. By 1966 seven groups had a total membership of 3625; 151 preprints were being sent out every month with an estimated total of 1·5 million copies per year. Potentially further growth might have been large: an estimated 200 groups might have been formed with ultimate costs as high as $10 million a year.

Though these preprints had been intended to be informal memoranda, most of them were publications—often being succeeded shortly afterwards by the substantive papers. This wasteful duplicate publication for some articles together with the poor scientific quality of others led correspondents to *Science* to advocate ending the experiment—which was done (126–8). A similar debate occurred with a proposal by the American Psychological Association for an early dissemination scheme of unedited and unreviewed manuscripts, one psychologist fearing that the system would become 'a vast sewer carrying garbage from one scientist to another', and the scheme was abandoned (129).

Hence it is not likely that serious scientists would remain content with any future system that lumped their papers together with a lot of junk.

Some sort of evaluation is inescapable; what is all important is how it is practised: internal or external, how many referees and of what type, what checks and appeal mechanisms, and so on. Even if largely anecdotal, we now have a fund of experience of the workings and effects of peer review, and the last three chapters have examined its benefits and dangers. Let us now turn the discussion around and look at the characteristics of science; what can peer review tell us about science (including medicine) and can we improve our assessments by making better use of the scientific method?

Such an examination might seem artificial. Science is the process of advancing knowledge, asking questions, and testing hypotheses, whereas peer review is the process of assessing how well an individual study matches up to the scientific ideal. Yet if scientists have a duty to do research they also have an obligation to expose it to general appraisal—which means publication. Ziman's 'The object of science is publication' (46) may be an exaggeration, but it emphasizes the duty that scientists have to publish good quality articles regularly throughout their career.[1] And if high quality articles predicate peer review, then the latter is part of the wider concept of science and is not so much a different category as might be thought.

CHARACTERISTICS OF SCIENTISTS AND SCIENCE

Scientists are trained by apprenticeship, learning that research is a social activity with highly critical standards (both internal and external) which should lead to continual self-correction (130). From a social scientist's point of view, science is said to show universalism, organized scepticism, communality, humility, and disinterestedness (53). Recently, also, science has shown publicly that it is self-policing. At first it was slow to react to the spate of reports about piracy, plagiarism, and forgery (100), but official bodies have now agreed on how to act over new examples—for example, the recommendations by Harvard or the Association of American Medical Colleges (131,132).[2]

FOUR PHASES OF SCIENCE

There are several views on how science progresses, but the one I find the easiest to accommodate sees development occurring in four main phases (46). Firstly, all is vagueness, mystery, and conjecture. The second phase is discovery, giving rise to new observations, which are objective and repeatable. The third phase, breakthrough, leads to a general pattern of explanation, and the fourth, classic, fills in the remaining pieces of the jigsaw. As Kuhn has pointed out, at any one time the climate of professional opinion may be as important as the genius of individuals in determining the intellectual history of a subject (134).

FIRST PHASE (VAGUENESS AND CONJECTURE)

In the first phase of science few scientists can be expected to accept a thesis without being able to validate it: they need data rather than will-o-the-wisp speculations. On the other hand, articles that generate hypotheses may be just as (or even more) important as articles that prove or confirm hypotheses. The difficulty of peer review is to spot the ones that are likely to be winners. Nevertheless, some journals are generous towards speculations, and may have large sections for these (making it clear that they are just that) and a few journals will print them as Letters to the Editor.

Relman agrees with a correspondent to the *New England Journal of Medicine* (135) that without peer review scientific letters may be published with unrecognized flaws (though his are subjected to internal assessment by his hanging committee, with only 25 per cent being accepted). Even so, in his view to apply a uniform review policy would sacrifice a valuable feature of a general weekly journal: the rapid dissemination of new ideas and observations. Hence Letters to the Editor should be reserved for very brief observations that can stand on their own or preliminary studies that will require follow-up. I can't agree with him: given that letters are usually included in data bases, such as *Index Medicus* and *Current Contents*, scientific articles that have not received rigorous external assessment may mislead the casual reader who knows nothing of editorial policy. For these reasons the *BMJ* has a section entitled 'Unreviewed Reports' (which are nevertheless discussed by our hanging committee) for anecdotes or speculations based on slim data where these can be printed under their true colours. These are recorded in the *BMJ* index but do not appear in the *Index Medicus*.

Finally, some journals are now entirely devoted to speculations and hypotheses, though even these use peer review, having a rejection rate of 50 per cent.

Often, of course, a topic never progresses beyond the first stage. Every editor will have encountered a theory that is plausible, based on no data but put over with vigour by a committed and honest research worker, often dealing with a condition that arouses strong emotions—in medicine, for example, the cause or treatment of cancer or multiple sclerosis is a top favourite. Sometimes the editor and the referee feel that the benefits of publication outweigh the risks. Often, however, they feel that the new theory is wrong: to accept it might do harm by raising false hopes; to reject it might be better but would provoke a charge of cowardice or supressing valuable advances.

Faced with the dilemma posed by some hypothesis-generating articles, I have been helped by the guidance provided by Langmuir about how to recognize 'pathological science', such as extrasensory perception or flying saucers (table XIV) (136).

SECOND PHASE (DISCOVERY)

The second phase is the most challenging to the scientific community, because the new discovery (which is now supported by data) does not accord with the paradigm, the current orthodoxies. Initially articles reporting such findings are likely to be submitted to one of the élite core journals, often to a general one (such as *Nature* or *Science*, or the *Lancet* or the *BMJ*), which are widely read, publish rapidly, and have a broad coverage. They have also been said to be run by and for the establishment (136); whatever this charge means, all these journals have high rejection rates, and inevitably they will decline some articles that turn out to be world shakers.

If the authors then seek publication in a specialty archival journal (or seek it initially without submitting their article to a general journal), they are likely to find that the response depends on the discipline. Zuckerman and Merton interpreted such variations in rejection rates, which were confirmed by Gordon's research, in three ways: firstly, by the different consensus between referees for 'hard' and 'soft'

Table XIV. Features of pathological science.

The maximum effect observed is produced by causative agent of barely detectable intensity.

The magnitude of the effect is substantially independent of the intensity of the cause.

The effect is of a magnitude that remains close to the limits of detectability, or many measurements are necessary because of the very low statistical significance of the results.

There are claims of great accuracy; there are fantastic theories contrary to experience.

Direct criticisms, given in person, are met by ad hoc excuses thought up on the spur of the moment.

The ratio of supporters to critics rises up to somewhere near to 50 per cent and then gradually falls to nil.

---

science; second, the decision patterns for the various disciplines; and, third, the amount of space available for publication (5,36).

The first aspect, consensus levels, has already been considered (p. 69); The second Gordon examined in the light of the suggestion (5) that in journals with high rejection rates the decision rule was: 'when in doubt, reject', and in ones with low rates: 'when in doubt, accept'. He confirmed this theory for specialist medical journals, finding that more assessment was used for an article to be accepted by a journal with a high rejection rate than by one with a low rate. For general medical journals, however, obviously other factors came into decision-making; Gordon found that their editors were concerned to pick out papers with general interest. For these reasons the two types of editors chose referees with different characteristics. Specialist journal editors wanted an expert, somebody at the top of his subject; general journal editors wanted a knowledgeable expert who could place the findings in the perspective needed for a general readership.

Gordon also found that specialist medical journal editors were inherently cautious, preferring to take few risks.[3] So possibly medical researchers hold different professional and intellectual values from biological researchers, he commented, and opt for a conservative approach. If his thesis is true (and I suspect it mostly is), I find this timidity by editors of specialist medical journals surprising; surely a specialist reader is better placed to judge the merits of a way out article for himself, and here above all there is scope for an editor to indulge in what Michael O'Donnell has called 'editorial irresponsibility'—occasionally forgetting fairness, balance, and so on, flinging caution to the winds and publishing an article on a hunch that it may be true and important, whatever his advisers say.[4]

Why are there limitations to the traditional open-mindedness of the scientist? One list (137) includes: cultural blinding factors, methodological conceptions, thinking in terms of substantive models, resistance to the usefulness of mathematics, religious beliefs, patterns of social interaction (snobbery), pattern of specialization, and poor refereeing. The last of these has been emphasized by Yalow, who won a Nobel Prize for her work on radio-immunoassay: 'the truly imaginative are not being judged by their peers. They have none!' Her original article was rejected by *Science* and initially by the *Journal of Clinical Investigation*. Her Nobel Prize essay (138) contains part of the *JCI's* initial letter of rejection and she comments that a compromise with the editors (including the apparently trivial insistence on leaving out 'insulin antibody' from the title) eventually resulted in acceptance (139).

Ruderfer has provided details of another 'erroneous rejection', of a paper dealing with atomic time-keeping which he claims corrected a published dispute. He ascribes the rejection to referees who were over-preoccupied with theory. Of the four of the nine reviews of his article available for discussion, one lacked scientific rigour, another did not justify the statements made, another refused to discuss the issues, while the last contained two major errors (140).

Matthew effect
At this second stage the Matthew effect is likely to operate.

Reviewers and editors are more likely to believe work by an author who is known than by one who is not; after all, the former has more to lose if his work is wrong and he has probably had more opportunities for expert review by colleagues before he submits his article for publication (139).[5]

That some resistance by scientists to scientific discovery is inevitable does not mean that resistance is commoner than acceptance in science, or that scientists are no less open-minded than other men (140). On the contrary, objectivity is greater and resistance is less than in other walks of life, and in medicine, for example, devices such as the random-ized double-blind controlled trial have been introduced to prevent the intrusion of personal bias (141). Nevertheless, scientists should recognize that such resistance occurs, particularly to novelty (134), and try to understand it.

How much harm does initial rejection by a major general or specialist archival journal cause? The invisible colleges are likely to know of the findings already (142), the scientist or his colleagues will be performing further studies to confirm or modify them, and these days he is likely to achieve publication somewhere, thereby achieving some validation and personal priority. I don't believe that today a brilliant paper such as the one by Waterston (p. xi) could remain unpublished for so long.[6]

Self-publication

Nevertheless, some workers have even had to publish their work themselves. *The Thorny Way of Truth (documents on the process of restoration of the absolute space-time conceptions)* by Stefan Marinov goes even further than this: a fascinating collection of 'representative' exchanges of letters with journal editors, it contains detailed arguments about his radical approach (143). Few people outside the subject, I suspect, could understand more than the general drift of these, but, as *Nature* commented in reviewing the book (144), its 285 pages show that to refuse publication without providing justification does less than justice to an author and plays into the hands of the conspiracy theorists—adding that those responsible for journals or funding bodies will note with disquiet that the more conscientious they are, the more conscientious a reply they will probably receive.

This supports one point well made by Ruderfer. In ordinary aspects of our society there are mechanisms for correcting major errors: the law courts, ombudsmen, and sports referees. Against possibly faulty peer review, on the other hand, there is no statutory right of appeal (140).

He then goes on to make a number of recommendations. No decision should be taken when disputes remain unresolved. All reviewers' comments should be subject to possible publication. The possibility of classifying manuscripts from evolutionary to revolutionary should be considered. In any dispute the assessor should be regarded as a contestant rather than a referee. Reviewers should be required to indicate the changes necessary for acceptance. The boundary of the dispute should be narrowed. An appeal mechanism should be developed. The editor should publish data on reviewing. Finally, the possibility of developing professional reviewers should be considered.[7]

Some of these suggestions are discussed in the chapter on improving peer review, but most of them are more relevant to an ivory tower than to a workaday journal office. In the end publication is a privilege and not a right. Most journals are run on a shoestring. Most referees are hard-working unpaid anonymous expert volunteers in the scientific process (and spend from a few hours to up to a day of their spare time in assessing an individual article (146,147)'). And most editors agonize about the risks to the reputation of their journals if they are known consistently to turn down good work. There is a limit to the amount of to-ing and fro-ing that is tolerable and with the likelihood that all articles can now get published somewhere a time comes when both sides must agree to disagree. What these published case histories have shown me is how far editors and advisers are prepared to go in reconsidering articles, with or without ripostes from the author and further judgments from uncommitted referees.

Parallels: peer review, science, and medicine

Errors in decisions

Inevitably some errors will occur. Small reported on a major one in his survey of 4203 papers in chemistry that were cited more than ten times a year (87). Even Yalow admits, however, that she has never failed to publish her worthwhile papers eventually and that sometimes she has come to appreciate the reviews she had initially resented (139).

The classic story to tell here is the so-called rejection in 1937 by *Nature* of the paper by (Sir) Hans Krebs reporting his 'citric acid' cycle (as he liked to call it (148)). In fact, the letter from the journal regretted only that the editor had sufficient letters for six or seven weeks, stating that if Krebs did not mind the delay the editor would keep it hoping to use it (instead, Krebs sent it off within two weeks to the journal *Enzymologia* in Holland, which published it within two months) (149).

Finally, a few of the complaints about the unfairness of peer review relate to papers about non-science which are never heard of again. The difficulties that editors and referees face are well underlined by Ziman: 'By his contempt for the current consensus, by his condemnation of all accepted theories and his insistence that he alone is favoured with the true light, the author puts himself outside of the scientific community and beyond scholarly observations' (46).

THIRD PHASE (BREAKTHROUGH)

In the third phase of a scientific revolution, breakthrough, everybody has suddenly come to accept the thesis and wants to climb on the bandwagon. Here different sets of problems arise for peer review. Theoretically at this stage scientists can apply their full criteria to judging their colleagues' discoveries. These will include, firstly, explanatory value (such as generality, span of relevance, and rank in the general hierarchy of explanation) and, second, their clarifying power (the degree to which these judgments resolve what has hitherto been perplexing. The third set of criteria (in this view, which is that of Sir Peter Medawar

81

(150)) include the originality in the research, the surprisingness of the solution to the problem, the elegance of the solution, the economy of thought and work, and the size (and difficulty) of the enterprise as a whole. 'The scientist values research by the size of its contribution to that huge logically articulated structure of ideas which is already, though not yet half built, the most glorious accomplishment of mankind'.

From Medawar's encomium we might think that all was well, even if self-evidently some contributions are larger than others. Nevertheless, by now the scientific paper does not stand alone: it is embedded in the literature of the subject. Moreover, it is not the final word but a contribution —one of the bricks from which the whole edifice is built. The key questions for the referees to answer are whether the brick has already been laid by somebody else, how big the building should be, and how many bricks are needed to complete the foundations and the ground floor. Thus recently complaints have increased not only about the proliferation of the scientific literature but also about unnecessary fragmentation. Theoretically peer review ought to be able to encourage one (evolution) but prevent the other (unrestrained and pointless proliferation)—or at least contain it.

Proliferation of publications

Complaints about the proliferation of published material are hardly new. In 1899 in his presidential address to the physiology section of the British Association, J. N. Langley (later professor of physiology at Cambridge) complained that the scientist was being restricted to a narrower and narrower specialism. Nor was this the whole of his burden: 'Much that he is forced to read consists of records of defective experiments, confused statements of wearisome descriptions of detail, and unnecessarily protracted discussion of unnecessary hypotheses. The publication of such matter is a serious injury to the man of science; it absorbs the scanty funds of his libraries, and steals away his poor hours of leisure' (151).

In a lecture given forty years later, just after the start of the second world war, Sir Robert Hutchison also complained of the bulk of the medical literature: on average two articles about tuberculosis had been published every day for the first forty years of the century (152). Science, he thought, was in danger of suffocating in its own secretions, and Britain should have only one general medical journal and one specialist journal for each discipline. And almost another forty years later another commentator pointed out that for over sixty years the *Index Medicus* had weighed 2 kg; between 1946 and 1955, however, its mass had risen to 4 kg and from 1956 to the time of writing (1978) to 30 kg (153). At this rate the *Cumulated Index Medicus* for 1985 would weigh 1000 kg, being contained in over 200 volumes.[8]

Finally, Waksman had described the harm produced by the information explosion: a decreased availability of journals, a decreasing value of the journal contents, and the burial of new ideas in the discussion section of the article (32).

Number of authors

Another cause for comment has been the number of authors per article. Between 1886 and 1977 the proportion of single-author papers fell from 98·5 to 4 per cent. The number of authors in major articles in the *Lancet* and the *New England Journal of Medicine* over the years rose, respectively, from a mean per paper of 1·3 and 1·2 in 1930 to 4·3 and 4·2 in 1975 (154). Such proliferation seemed to be confined to the classic medical weeklies, for the other general journals and journals in the basic sciences and applied psychology all had significantly fewer authors per article. Did this difference reflect multidisciplinary research? Whatever the answer, if current trends continued, by the year 2076 each of these medical journals would have at least 24 authors per article.

The view that the increase in the number of articles, authors per article, and journals (which now may number 100,000 for science and 20,000 for biomedicine) is a sign of disease in the scientific community has not gone unchallenged. De Solla Price has shown that for over 300 years scientific publications have grown steadily by 6–7 per cent every year (15). His rule of thumb is that a scientist who publishes one article every year can absorb the contents of more than one other paper per month, but less than one a day. This leads to a few hundred individuals keeping each other in business—the same size as the membership of the early scientific societies and of today's invisible colleges.

Disciplines tend to split every ten years or so (155) and the new subdisciplines do not necessarily correspond with the organizational and professional structures—which are slower to alter than the way in which the pattern of new knowledge changes. Authors, Solla Price concludes, write for a small audience of peers and count themselves successful if the latter read these articles and build on them. Each paper will be built on four or five predecessors, with about half its references to these, with the other half being miscellaneous (historical allusions, flattery, and so on).

Health or disease?

Two other thoughtful commentators have joined the debate on whether more means worse. Ziman is another who thinks that the growth of scientific publications may be a natural consequence of scientific progress—a sign of health rather than disease (156). Yet he does not spare the mass of unoriginal publications stored in the archives which are characterized by the triviality of the results, the incompetence of the experimental methods, or the purely technological or commercial context in which the findings are reported. And Waksman has complained that an ever-higher proportion of published work is concerned with details rather than with principles. The result is that the value of any individual journal has decreased drastically (32).

Objectively, Waksman's accusation has been supported by surveys finding that only 10–14 per cent of authors write up their work to contain useful information (157), by consensus analysis in which experts have judged that only

10–15 per cent of articles are important (158), and by citation analysis disclosing that between a quarter and a half of articles are never used as a reference after publication (86). Finally, a large amount of fragmentation or duplication of publication goes on. The findings of a single study are often spread among several journals or even published in identical or slightly modified forms in different journals or books (159).

Everybody must decide for himself whether the gravamen of excessive publication has been proved or not. My own view is that it has and that the lack of citation of so many articles confirms this; stopping it must be a priority. The problem may not be the same for all disciplines: thus an analysis of publications on schistosomiasis concludes that there has been an 'author explosion' rather than a 'literature explosion' (160). Some element of information explosion is necessary, indeed vital, but there is no shortage of methods to cope with this—including more and better abstracts, review articles and journals, new types of knowledge bases (such as the interesting experiment of the hepatitis knowledge base (161,162)),[9] and computerized retrieval services.

For current awareness, working scientists still give journals priority over discussions with colleagues, *Current Contents*, abstracts, or on-line computer services (163). Hence improving the standards of journals is obviously important—in particular, emphasis on true originality, scientific reliability, and the importance of any article they receive. Nevertheless, for journals with medium to high rejection rates peer review's main role is of a traffic policeman, diverting the poorer articles away from journals of high repute to those of lower repute (p. 5). If authors go on trying they will get their articles published somewhere.

Journals reflect the prevailing ethos of the scientific community and hence the priority must be to change this. The obvious alteration that is needed is to judge the worth of individuals by looking at the quality of their research rather than the quantity of articles this gives rise to.

Emphasis on quality

More and more commentators are now echoing lack of emphasis on quality. The Harvard guidelines for avoiding fraud, for example, criticize the practice of publishing small batches of research findings in several different publications, rather than concentrating on one major publication (131). Berry (164) and Angell (143) have observed that too little weight is attached to the scientific merit of a paper or to the journal of publication. A publication in one of the top journals with a vigorous policy should be equivalent to several publications elsewhere. Nevertheless, I have been told privately that academics aiming at senior appointments are even now being advised by their Deans to publish much more, putting their names on as many articles as possible. A rating system for promotions whereby a single-author article scores 1 point, a dual-author article half a point, and so on, with 15 points being needed, say, for promotion to a readership, is one of the causes of multi-author publications. Surely we can do better than this?

A suggestion that I favour is one to curtail the number of papers that a scientist may cite in his curriculum vitae. The current glut of articles would almost certainly be curtailed if this was restricted to ten (165), and in any case the number should be related to the grade of post (166). Should we go further: asking an applicant to list the three articles he considers the best in a year (113), or, even more radically, limit the number of publications by each author to five per year or 50 papers or books in his lifetime (with multiple authorship of whatever number counting as half a publication) (153)?

The last proposal was criticized heavily in the subsequent correspondence (167–170), one writer complaining that it was more in the realms of humour than a serious contribution since it ignored scholarly research into the proliferation of the scientific literature. Few would deny, however, that some aspects of this proliferation are alarming. Even if many articles do little harm because they are unread and uncited, the costs to the community of the research and writing up, peer review and subediting, printing and distribution, and library catologuing and storage are enormous—to say nothing of the danger that the important may be buried by the trivial.

Just as serious, however, is what the proliferative process tells us about the attitudes and credulity of the scientific community. Though scientists destined to gain the Nobel Prize come to deliberately restrict the number of articles they publish, concentrating on quality rather than quantity (54), the scientific community in general evaluates achievement by numbers of contributions rather than their content—giving credit to so-called productivity.

Thus John Darsee was widely regarded as a brilliant researcher, 'charismatic' and 'exceptionally able'. During his training period at Emory University from 1974 to 1979 he was co-author of no fewer than 10 full-length papers and 45 abstracts, and at Harvard of 50 articles and abstracts; the computer print-out of the 241 papers citing his work was over 29 feet long (171). Yet surely somebody, somewhere, at some stage should have come to the obvious conclusion: work of such weight, intricacy, and diversity was impossible. Instead, Darsee was judged on apparent achievement on grounds that seemingly ignored the content.

In the discussion on scientific fraud at the 1985 meeting of the American Association for the Advancement of Science speaker after speaker spoke of the excessive attention paid to prolific publishing as a measure of significant achievement in promotion and funding decisions: 'academic promotions committees count and weigh papers; they do not read them'. Several highly publicized cases of scientific fraud had taken place in laboratories where there was a great deal of publishing, far above the norm (172). Woolf estimated the mean number of papers published by each scientist as less than 10 a year. In the five years preceding Summerlin's resignation after falsifying an experiment with mice (100), his chief, Robert Good, had published an average of 68 papers a year. In the five years before Darsee's resignation his chief, Eugene Braunwald, had published an average of 28·5 a year. In the five years before the dismissal of Vijay Soman, who fabricated data and plagiarized a paper (p. 52), his chief, Philip Felig, had published an average of almost 32 papers a year.

Whether pressures to publish are responsible for the more serious cases of fraud remains unknown (17). Nevertheless, some comments on the conditions at the Harvard Laboratory—'hurried pace and emphasis on productivity and limited interaction with senior scientists' (173)—remind me in a different connection of the impossible lives politicians are expected (or expect themselves) to lead. The description of Anthony Crosland's last few days alive is horrifying (174): apart from his routine duties as Foreign Secretary and Member of Parliament, he was up most of the night at a Brussels EEC meeting on Tuesday; in London with a dinner party (where he made a speech) on Wednesday; morning Cabinet meeting, evening divisions at the House of Commons on Thursday; visit to art exhibition, dinner and after dinner seminar at Oxford on Friday; work on speeches on detente and Rhodesia in his cottage on Saturday and Sunday, when he had his final stroke.

FOURTH PHASE (CLASSIC)

So an emphasis on quality should be a priority in stopping the unnecessary proliferation of scientific publications, and as a result of his specialist knowledge the referee's advice is crucial. This emphasis is particularly important for the fourth phase of the scientific discovery, fitting in the remaining parts of the jigsaw. More than at any other stage, here scientists tend to do 'Brownian motion' research (112), and peer review has a vital role in distinguishing between the useful and the useless.

In a striking comparison, the exponential proliferation of the medical literature has been likened to schistosomiasis (160) (figure 5). The definitive host remains the same (man), the miracidium equals the manuscript, and the environment (the water) is the library. The number of the intermediate hosts (journals) must exceed a threshold for an epidemic to start, and this can be controlled in two ways: firstly, by decreasing the numbers of articles attacking the host, and, second, by ensuring that these have a high virulence (quality).

Parallels: peer review, science, and medicine

The lessons for peer review are obvious. In particular, editors and reviewers must not be coerced by current pressures for publishing snippets of information very fast into abandoning one of their main preoccupations, with quality. Stossel has described how the 'arms race' for very rapid publication (within a week or two) of trendy research by quality journals has serious implications for the scientific community: it increases the pressure on all journals to accelerate their rate of paper processing; it means that editors begin to redefine what is normal behaviour among scientists; it increases the burden on reviewers; it encourages fragmentation of publications; and it undermines the value of prepublication for determining priority and providing a preliminary review of scientific work. Moreover, the demand for rapid peer review exposes the referee to a conflict of interest: if a competitor's work is worthy of publication within a week then, by implication, the reviewer's work invites the same treatment. Not to go along with the system is to risk lack of reciprocal treatment.

Even though over 60 per cent of scientists have had the experience once of somebody else publishing an article on similar work first—and 17 per cent more than twice—Stossel's poll of 22 prestigous scientists (including 11 Nobel laureates and 16 members of the National Academy of Science), all of whom replied, showed that few thought that rapid publications had influenced their rise to prominence (175).

In all the suggestions for emphasizing quality rather than quantity a sense of humour and the personal approach should not be forgotten, particularly when the author is senior enough to know better. I wish more scientists would be as frank as Max Delbruck was when he wrote to Mrs Seymour Benzer (54):

Dear Dotty,
   Please tell Seymour to stop writing so many papers. If I gave them the attention his papers *used* to deserve, they would take all my time. If he *must* continue, tell him to do what Ernest Mayr asked his mother to do in her long daily letters—namely, underline what is important.

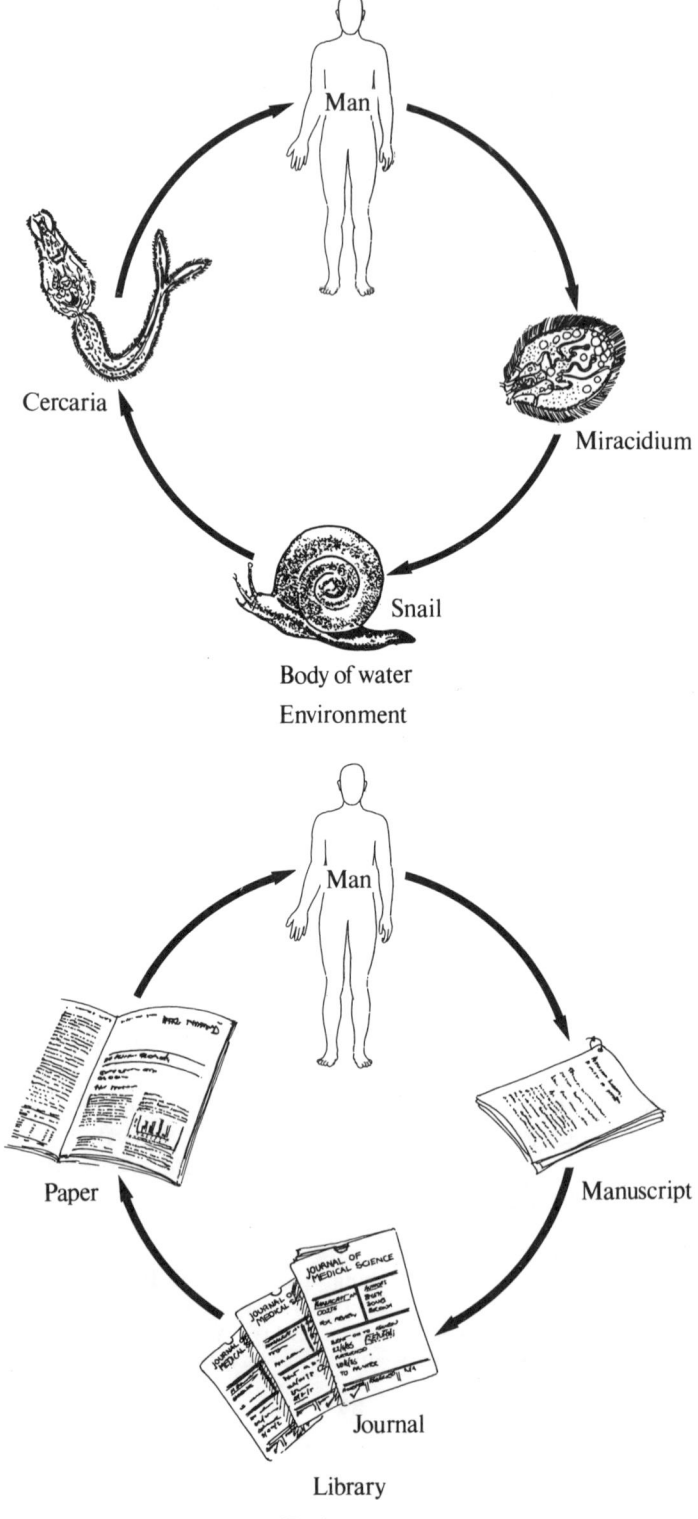

Man

Cercaria

Miracidium

Snail

Body of water

Environment

Man

Paper

Manuscript

JOURNAL OF MEDICAL SCIENCE

Journal

Library

Environment

Having examined what peer review might do in the various stages how does science itself fare if we look at it in the light of the accusations made against peer review?

Douglas-Wilson accused peer review of being slow, tending to élitism and conservatism, and having a potential for bigotry (176). Scientific evolution may be slow, often because scientists are unprepared for substantial shifts from the paradigm—whether in 'Normal Science', such as most of the discoveries in medicine, or 'Revolutionary Science', such as the discoveries of a Lavoisier or an Einstein (134). Elitist and conservative are charges that can be supported by some episodes: 'Long built his [career] out of little more than élitism . . . the power of the élite bore Long aloft for a decade, and would doubtless have carried him much further but for his single miscalculation of placing forged data under Quay's scrutiny' (100). Nevertheless, science is concerned with questioning, testing, and abandoning old hypotheses and, as shown by the continual fragmentation of the invisible colleges into new ones, any conservatism may be more apparent than real, reflecting official standpoints rather than true ones.

The last of Douglas-Wilson's accusations, a tendency to bigotry, I would suggest is untrue of science as a whole, even though it may apply to a few individuals or departments, particularly about a subject where no clear consensus has been established. The mechanism for avoiding all these hazards is free communication among scientists—both verbal (formal and informal) and written. And such free communication must include journal editors as well. Bizarre theories such as those on plant genetics held by Lysenko, who terrorized the agriculturalists in the Soviet Union in the Stalinist era, can survive only where all channels of communication have been blocked—Gustafson, for instance, has commented on the current insistence of Soviet hosts to American visitors that they believe in deferring to

FIGURE 5. Comparison between the cycles of schistosomiasis and medical literatures. (Reproduced from Warren and Goffman (160) by kind permission of the authors and publishers).

the skills of the experts and not venturing subjective opinions outside their own specialty (177).

This, then, is the difficult balance that peer review for journals has to try to ensure—between scientific rigour and freedom of discussion. In particular, it still has much to learn from the continually self-correcting nature of science (178). It might also learn much from the experience of peer review for other purposes (such as research grants). This is the theme of the next chapter.

7

Correlations: lessons for editorial peer review from other types

Correlation (1562). *Mutual relation of two or more things (implying intimate or necesary connection).*

Referees for journal articles are one form of 'status judges', who play an integral part in controlling social systems (5). Other examples include teachers; members of panels for deciding on appointments, awards and honours, and elections to prestigious learned societies; critics in the arts; and assessors for applications for research grants. The activities of the last resemble those for editorial peer review. Do the rhetoric and data that have accumulated throw any light on peer review for learned journals?

Increasingly most scientific research is now funded by outside bodies (179). In chemistry, for example, the acknowledgements in articles in the *Journal of the Chemical Society* show that, though in 1910 only 10 per cent of research was funded externally, in 1925 the proportion was 50 per cent and in 1975, 78 per cent. Until the late 1960s probably most worthy research proposals were eventually funded, and few complaints were published about the general allocation system (180). Recently, however, because of the increased amount of research and its costs, as well as static or diminishing funds, it has become likely that the Medical Research Council will be able to fund less than half the first-rate applications from universities (181). (A few of the sums are now enormous: for example, the annual budget of CERN, the high-energy physics establishment outside Geneva, is currently $300m (182)).

Ironically today one form of peer review may be allowing a research worker to publish his findings, while another

Notes begin on p. 150. References begin on p. 160.

form may be denying the same work the opportunity to progress by refusing him a research grant (183). As a result, complaints about how funds are allocated have increased from both scientists and politicians, some research has been started, and some changes have been proposed.

EVALUATION

Evaluation follows similar lines for most applications for research grants. Each proposal goes to the staff secretary in the nearest discipline, who chooses knowledgeable reviewers, asking them about the application's merits. Often if the report is totally unfavourable from all the assessors, a director rejects the application on his own responsibility, or, if the reviewers disagree fundamentally, he seeks the opinion of others.

Usually, however, the forms and opinions go to a board for a decision. This scores the application on a scale, and whether the researcher gets a grant or not depends on the cut-off point at the time. For example, at one time the Medical Research Council could fund most applications that scored 3·5 or more (on a scale of 1–6); in 1985 this figure was raised to 4·0, and some applicants are now being told that their research programme has been approved but cannot be funded.

Variations

There are many variations (major and minor) on this so-called single-panel peer review. Some research agencies with well-defined objectives reject a project straight away without peer review because it does not fall within the scope of these or is self-evidently of poor quality. The number of referees asked usually varies between two and five (sometimes more in the USA) and they are chosen widely, in much the same way as those for journals. If the subject is outside the referee's own experience, he or she is encouraged to suggest a suitable alternative.

The forms used have a four-point or a five-point scale and ask questions about originality, potential value of the research, appropriateness of the design, suitability of the methods, and feasibility within the time proposed—as well as the applicant's standing. Another question often asked is about the ability of the principal investigator. Finally most forms have space for supplementary general or detailed comments.

The board may take its final decision with or without knowing who the referees were, information which may be contained in an accompanying sealed envelope. Nevertheless, it is unusual to blind the referees to the applicant's identity. Several commentators have argued that this would be impossible without distorting the project and destroying its integrity (184,185), or that it is undesirable.

Feedback

A major difference among grant-giving bodies is the amount of information provided to unsuccessful applicants. In the USA under the Freedom of Information Act feedback has become the rule (186). Elsewhere, however, it is rare to provide them with detailed reasons for the decision (although sometimes this is done—for example, for applications that are deferred, or when the agency wishes the applicant to concentrate on part of the proposal, and when advice might help in formulating new proposals).

The reasons for not giving any feedback are largely logistic and financial. Every year grant-giving agencies have a large number of applications for grants, of which a decreasing number can be funded (187)). From the experience in the USA, providing applicants with full reasons for rejections would need an estimated extra 20 per cent of funds. Since few research agencies will allow any appeal against the decision, they think that it is a logical to spend all the limited resources on funding research itself.

Agencies claim that they are protected against biased assessments in several ways. Firstly, their scientific programme directors are fully in touch with progress in the disciplines. Second, they use several assessors. Third, one of the members of the final selection committee is often nominated to go into the application very thoroughly and act as its advocate (or critic).

As an outsider, I find both sets of arguments *jejune*. Surely, given the amount of work that has gone into the application, by the scientist and the referees, the maximum value should be derived from the reports. And I would question the costs mentioned—haven't our research bodies heard of word-processors? Again, the idea of protection against bias seems insecurely based: once a scientist works in an office his grasp of day-to-day advances is bound to fall off, as I know from personal experience. Appeals against decisions are a nuisance, but should be part of the process. Surely one solution would be a controlled trial into both these important questions, a suggestion made by Sir Richard Doll (188).

Research

Research into peer review for research grants has been patchy. For outcome, the most that has been done in Britain is for the agencies to record in their regular reports the publications resulting from the research—though these lists are incomplete (189). There has been no categorization of publications into major or minor using citation analysis or the journal of publication. In the USA, on the other hand, a few studies have used citation analysis as a measure of outcome (22,190). No attempt seems to have been made anywhere to analyze the fate of rejected applications, and, if these were funded elsewhere, to compare their outcome with the outcome of the accepted projects.

In Britain the analysis of the peer review process for research grants has been limited to measuring consensus among the assessors. In the USA, on the other hand, as a result of concern by scientists and, particularly, politicians about unfairness in allocating funds, a major research project has been undertaken. Its results are reassuring—though these cannot be applied to all research agencies, in either the USA or Britain. These are discussed later, but first let us consider some of the accusations made against peer review for research grants and the suggestions for improving it.

CRITICISMS AND PROPOSALS

Horrobin has long been a persistent critic of the system, for both grants and journal articles—describing peer review as a philosophically faulty concept which is disastrous for science (114), and assessors and research administrators as barriers to scientific research (191,192). The real power lies with the research administrator, who can manipulate the system to sink a good application or encourage a bad one (a suggestion also supported by Michie (193)). In Horrobin's experience about one in five assessors' reports contains a major error (documented for his own work) and peer review has a built-in bias against highly innovative work. In particular, there are often only two or three sources of research grants, all of which are likely to use the same reviewers.

The solution, Horrobin suggests, is to allocate research money partly as a block grant to the university department according to the number of students and partly as a grant to the individual academic (194). Instead of the 'failed expert' allocating the funds, another possibility is that a new form of committee should be responsible. The latter would be composed of three types of people: laymen with an interest in research for personal reasons[1]; doctors, such as general practitioners, who confront disease as it really is; and successful businessmen used to dealing with expert advice. The amount of money given to any research group shall be strictly limited, and the evaluative criteria include the following: (a) the record of recent research; (b) the presence of considerable uncertainty; (c) high-risk projects where the outcome matters; and (d) likely immediate practical effects.

Another attack on present day research funding and peer review (196) has concluded that the latter will have to change. Currently, this argues, the system has at least six major flaws. Firstly, new ideas cannot be protected from the reviewers. Second, creative science is difficult to evaluate because it is new. Third, the only way to write a research grant application is to describe experiments that have already been done. Fourth, the correct evaluation of data as these are produced is very difficult. Fifth, it is difficult to appeal against a negative decision. Sixth, and finally, the system favours those who write well.

Since other branches of human activity have professional reviewers (again, the example of dramatic and music critics is given), it is suggested that similar professional independent review panels should be developed for research funding.

NOT SO DISTANT ECHOES

Some of these charges and suggestions have been echoed by others—in particular, the lack of any appeal and the possibility of plagiarism by referees; thus rivals should not review grant applications (183). Three suggestions for improving the system are to base grants on departments, to base them on productivity, or to improve the existing system—with an emphasis on signed reviews, productivity, fairer reporting, and an appeals procedure.

The referee's judgment should be supported by documented evidence; even charges such as triviality, irrelevance, and general lack of understanding can all be documented (117). The peer review system has been said to be worse for grant proposals than for journals: opinions take two or three times as long to come and are more often ill-formed and damaging; moreover, it is harder to argue with a grant agency than with a journal. Finally, this critic argues that the aim should be to establish a fair system of peer review for grant proposals. If this was shown to work its details could be immediately adopted by editors as well.

Most of the issues were ventilated in the correspondence columns of *Science* after the publication of some proposed alternatives to peer review for research funding. Based on a productivity formula, these had included the number of degrees awarded, the number of papers published, the amount of federal and state money awarded, and the amount of money given by industry (197).

Correspondents objected to the probable extreme concentration of power in the programme manager (198), as well as to the possibility that shorter, less important research papers would proliferate (199,200). Numbers could not be substituted for scientific judgment, different types of research needed different amounts of money (201)—and who would decide on the amount of the block granted to the university? (202) The present system allowed for a judgment of the quality of past performance and future promise, and was essential for maintaining the health of science (203).

One proposal was that, instead of developing an entirely new system without peer review at all, the present system should be restructured (204). Any alterations should include the following: cutting out redundancy within and between grant agencies; limiting the number of proposals an individual investigator can submit; cutting out the consultancy fee; establishing regional review panels (rather than having them all situated centrally, at Washington); performing fewer expensive site visits; and looking closely at individual research empires.

Riposting to all these comments, the author of the original proposals emphasized the need for flexibility in allocating research grants; 70 per cent of the overall sum should go to the principal investigators, 20 per cent to departments, and 10 per cent to institutions (205). There was no evidence that peer review is linked to the progress of science or that it can define or identify quality. The fundamentals of quantum mechanics, organic synthesis, and DNA structure had all been discovered without peer review; moreover, some of the principal research institutions in the USA supported basic research without peer review, relying on their judgment of the investigator's competence and track record. Peer review could not predict the quality of proposed research: it was difficult enough to judge that of completed research (as witness the disagreement among reviewers about articles submitted for publication). No study had been done to show that allocating funds by peer review had produced any better results than would have occurred by lottery.

RESEARCH STUDIES

Even if they are thoughtful and based on experience, most of these comments are anecdotal. The few rigorous objective studies of the process of peer review started at least ten years ago, but until recently these had been confined to the USA. In describing one such study Noble discusses the influence on judgments about the worth of applied research, especially 'policy' or evaluative studies (200). As long ago as 1970 a study had shown that only 10 per cent of 152 comprehensive evaluation projects funded by federal government agencies had met the minimum scientific standards. In his view, peer review needs strengthening in two ways. Firstly, the use of formal standards would guide panels, making the grounds for judgment explicit. Second, evaluation of applications for renewed funding would be easier by looking at completed research, determining whether this had answered specific questions.

In a study carried out for the Department of Health, Education, and Welfare, Noble asked 15 judges to rate six proposals in two ways. Firstly, globally—as a single overall assessment. Second, as a composite assessment based on 67 separate ratings of methods (such as design, sampling, statistics, checking, and reporting). Two additional variations on this pattern of single-panel peer review depended (*a*) on whether the panel members also assessed the projects before they met as a group, and (*b*) whether they talked to the principal investigator.

Noble found that both types of assessment were moderately effective, as shown by the consistency of the ratings. Possible bias was introduced, however, by both the variations. Consensus might be improved, he suggested, by assembling two groups of experts, one about methods and the other about the overall importance of the work, and then making them operate as adversaries. Certainly experts should be able to communicate with the principal investigator, but this should be indirect—possibly through the permanent staff of the funding agency. There was also a case for blinding the assessors to the applicant's identities.

CITATION ANALYSIS

Concluding, Noble proposed that the evaluation of finished research could guide not only its use but also the funding of new research—an approach used by Carter, who investigated the use of citation analysis as an objective measure (22). She examined all the programme project grants and a sample of the 747 research project grants awarded by the NIH in 1967, linking the priority scores given by the initial review panel (composed of expert scientists in the discipline) with the subsequent citations.

Carter found no evidence that peer review had been biased by knowledge of which medical school was applying for the grant. Next, the applications that had produced the most cited 5 per cent of the journal articles had received higher priority scores than average, both at the initial applications and at the application for their renewal. Usually the citation rate was more related to the priority score in the second application than to the score in the first one. These observations, she considered, show that the peer review system is flexible and that it can change its judgment of applications to reflect changes in merit. They also show how uncertain are the preliminary judgments about the scientific merits of proposed research.

The use of citation rates was also discussed by Gustafson, who concluded that the critics of peer review for research grants had yet to make their case (195). Of the National Science Foundations awards in chemistry, 80–85 per cent had gone to departments which had produced an average of over 60 citations per author over five years. The four or five departments which had received the lion's share of the grants had averaged about 400 citations per author.

Gustafson also examined the proposals for institutional funding, concluding that this might be the answer for large and co-ordinated programmes. For most types of fundamental research, however, the traditional project grant, with the priority partly determined by the worth of the other applications, was the best guarantee of scientific merit and accurate information. It was important to extend the existing safeguards: to choose advisers and agency staff who are representative of the best science; to limit their terms of service; to separate the evaluation of scientific merits from any consideration of the funds available; and to submit the entire system to periodic review and criticism.

Finally, he showed that the rank and file science advisers changed frequently, but these serving on the important policy committees did not. On the one hand, I find that the implications of this finding are reassuring: bias against a single project is unlikely to persist because of the prejudices of an individual assessor. On the other hand, there is the snag that policy is more likely to be static for some time, with a diminished potential for flexibility.

ROLE OF CHANCE

The most important analysis of peer review for research grants has come from Stephen and Jonathan Cole and Simon (207,208), who emphasize something that few other commentators have: the role of chance. Because of all the concerns expressed, they analyzed the process used by the National Science Foundation. The first phase of this research was based on 75 extended interviews with NSF staff, an analysis of 1200 proposals, and the reviewers' comments on 250 of these. The second phase was based on a re-evaluation by a new set of reviewers of 150 proposals for research grants.

For the first phase there were five main findings. Firstly, there was a high correlation between reviewer ratings and eventual fundings. Second, and unexpectedly, there was little correlation between the grants awarded and the previous scientific performance of the applicant (the number of papers published and citations). Third, reviewers from major institutions did not give preferential treatment to proposals from applicants at major institutions. Fourth, professional age had no strong relation to the ratings or the probability of receiving a grant. Fifth, and lastly, there was a low or moderate correlation beteween reviewer ratings and the following: rank of investigator in department; rank of department; geographical location; NSF funding history; and place of PhD training. From all this the Coles and Simon conclude that the NSF funding system was free from systematic bias.

In part two of their study they looked at 150 proposals covering three disciplines; half of these had been funded and half had not. They then had these proposals reviewed again by 12 other experts. The Coles and Simon came to three main conclusions. Firstly, the potential total number of reviewers for any proposal was at least 10—and probably over 20. Second, there was a moderately high correlation between the original NSF grading and that found in their study. Third, there was a reversal rate of 24–30 per cent, which was highest in the middle quintile of the original rankings but also occurred in the others; even the top quintile contained proposals that would not have been funded by the second assessment.

Other comments by the Coles and Simon are that their findings are unlikely to reflect different criteria between the two assessments, since both groups of reviewers were given identical instructions; the reviewers were drawn from the same population; and consensus among reviewers for anthropology and economics was no less than it was for the natural sciences. So, they conclude, the fate of a grant application is determined roughly half by the characteristics of a proposal and of the principal investigator and about half by 'the luck of the reviewer draw'—probably the result of real and legitimate differences of opinion about what good science is or should be. The reason why eminent scientists may be more likely to be funded than less well-known ones may be because they submit many proposals and are not put off by a single rejection.

PAST PERFORMANCE

One way to reduce the effect of chance, the Coles and Simon think, may be to give more weight to agreed criteria—for instance, the value of recently completed research rather than proposed work. This is one of several proposals for increased objectivity in scientific decision-making made by the members of the Science Policy Research Unit of the University of Sussex (laudably, they emphasize that the order of the authorship is on a rotating basis (119, 180,182,189,209)).

In the past, the unit members point out, there has been little attempt to use objective indicators, such as data on research output and past performance. Instead, the scientific community has relied almost entirely on qualitative peer review: 'the informed prejudices of wise men'. This method of allocating resources is in danger of breaking down, given the static budgets for research, the entrenchment of interests (particularly for so-called Big Science, such as radio-astronomy and high-energy physics), and the concentration of research activities in fewer and fewer institutions, and in an era of no growth it is an inefficient method of reconstructing scientific activity—particularly for identifying declining research topics and groups.

The unit's proposals for reforming and extending de-cision-making mechanisms fall into two parts. Firstly, obtaining more data on the inputs to scientific disciplines—how much is spent and how funds are allocated compared with other countries. Second, changing the peer review procedure, which, while it must remain the key factor in evaluation, needs major improvements—such as the use of foreign assessors, wider panels (including scientific 'laypeople'), and open evaluation systems in which the referee's opinion may be challenged.

THREE-STAGE EVALUATION

Some such changes have already been introduced in the Netherlands by the Organization for the Advancement of Pure Science (ZWO) (209). All proposals for research in physics are now judged by an ad hoc jury drawn from a range of disciplines, including chemists, mathematicians, and astronomers.

Evaluation takes place in three stages. In the first, members of the jury—who work by post, without communicating with one another—are sent the proposals and asked for questions and observations.

In the second, the applicant for the grant is sent these comments together with the anonymous opinions of six expert assessors (two of them from outside the Netherlands). These have been asked for reasons why the proposal is worthwhile or not—and not for a decision whether it should be accepted.

In the third, the jury uses the applicant's reply to grade the proposals on four criteria. The latter are: the ability of the researchers, the objectives of the work, the methods, and overall quality. Consensus among the members of the jury is high, and, though the decision rests with the ZWO board, it usually follows the jury's advice. The Dutch scientific community is said to be enthusiastic about this new procedure.[2]

'CONVERGING PARTIAL INDICATORS'

Finally, the Sussex unit has used a combination of several criteria—what they term 'converging partial indicators'—to assess the productivity, impact, and perceived importance of one Big Science project: the European Organization for Nuclear Research (CERN), compared with other similar projects (119). In intensive and structured interviews 182 experimental and high-energy physicists were asked to rank the linear accelerators at 14 different laboratories for their relative contributions to high-energy physics. Combined with other criteria (including citations), the results showed that for the resources invested all three US national laboratories had a better record than CERN. (The results of citation analysis, the unit found, had to be treated with some caution unless great care was taken to identify and allow for the 'mistaken' papers that appear during periods of theoretical uncertainty. Together with other indicators, however, its guarded use was valuable.)

LESSONS FOR JOURNALS

Can all these findings be applied to improving peer review for articles submitted to journals? Both senior science administrators and editors now recognize that new approaches are needed towards an old technique, even though no cogent reasons have been produced for abandoning expert assessment altogether.[3] Such changes, I suspect, will include more openness, the development of more explicit criteria, and more dialogue between the two sides (particularly comments by the authors on the referee's report before a decision is taken, together with an appeal mechanism.)

For difficult topics uncertainty may be reduced by using more assessors, within reasonable limits, which will vary with circumstances. Certainly I believe that a good case has been made for two practices: retaining the anonymity of the assessor and ceasing to ask him to make a recommendation about publication—which is the editor's decision, which he should take on a variety of grounds, of which the referee's report is just one.

For journals to adopt many of the measures proposed for allocating research funds would be expensive, time consuming, and, given the present day demands on the editor, possibly not feasible—though the next chapter discusses what improvements would be practicable. Unlike agencies giving research grants, journals have a fail-safe mechanism, in that most articles eventually get published; any unfairness is in the article's being rejected by the first journal or two of the authors' choice. This aspect was nicely caught in the leading article in *Science* commenting on its new editorial policy, which will not now consider appeals against its decision: 'each author of a returned manuscript can explain to his or her graduate students that "unfortunately we chose the week in which Darwin, Newton, Priestley, and Keynes submitted their own seminal discoveries"' (11).

Finally, one of the most valuable findings from these studies is that all processes may be 'unfair': they have a (largish) element of randomness. As the Coles and Simon point out, this may be unfortunate for the researcher, though it may have little impact on science as a whole.

(Whether funding agencies should reserve 5 per cent of their grants for zany projects, as has been suggested, so that the occasional unconventional project will bear fruit, is theoretically attractive but unlikely in the present era of cuts. On the other hand, editors could bear such a possibility in mind.)

In a way it is remarkable that the findings by the Coles and Simon should have provoked such surprise, for life itself has always been unfair and there are other examples of unfairness in science—scientists whose work has been ignored or even unpublished. The story of awards for the Nobel Prize illustrates the large random element to scientific recognition (54). Some scientists have failed to get the prize because their work was too early or was superseded after a war; others have got the prize for work that was subseqently shown to be wrong. In literature especially I am one of those who regret that the prize often seems to be awarded on political grounds rather than on pure merit and the omission of, say, Hemingway or Graham Greene is unfortunate.

Those true realists, the French, have signalled that unfairness is universal by introducing the concept of the 41st chair—whose occupants have failed to be selected to the Académie Francaise (which had 40 members). Its holders have included Déscartes, Molière, Rousseau, Flaubert, and Proust. So one lesson that we should all propagate is that, as in life in general, some arbitrariness in science is inevitable (for very sound reasons). Shouldn't recognition of this fact become part of scientific thinking?

8

Betterment: improving peer review

Betterment (1598). *Amendment, improvement, amelioration, reformation.*

Peer review, then, has many defects; some are inherent and have to be accepted, others are not and can be corrected. Given that the system has lasted for over 300 years, that to most of us totally free for all publication would be impracticable, and that surveys have shown that peer review is probably beneficial in 75–90 per cent of cases (as shown by the revision of articles according to the referee's suggestions), I believe that we should try to improve peer review before considering abandoning it.

Improvements can come from all three members of the triangle—author, editor, and referee—but the prime responsibility is the editor's. His priority should be to select and monitor his assessors, helping them to give adequate reviews with guidelines on what advice he needs and feedback about the eventual decision on the articles. Next he needs to make up his own mind about some important details of the process, including the number and type of referees for each article, blindness of assessment, signed reviews, and ripostes by the author. Finally the editor has to decide on his philosophy—whether to devise formats for suitable non-peer reviewed articles and whether his priority is to risk accepting articles that may be wrong or rejecting articles that may be right.

There is no consistent mechanism by which editors choose their assessors, though, like Benjamin Franklin's certainties, death and taxes, the certainty is that any assessor who provides a rapid, accurate, and helpful opinion is likely to be asked to repeat the performance again and again. A very few journals have even asked authors to nominate their own referee (211), and most editors will consider a request in reverse: not to ask a particular expert with whom the author may be in conflict.

Editors have some guidelines for assessing papers (for example, those issued by the Royal Society (33)), as have authors for writing them (for example, in articles or books on medical writing (212–17) or the 'Vancouver' recommendations (82), and, in particular, the journal's own 'Instructions to Authors'). Nevertheless, until recently the referee has had little guidance. Whimster has described his bewilderment at receiving an envelope containing an original article together with a brief and unhelpful letter from the *BMJ* asking for his opinion on its originality, scientific reliability, clinical importance, and suitability for that journal (218).

What the letter should also have contained, Whimster suggested in the light of experience, was a statement why he had been chosen as an assessor for the article; whether another referee was also being used (and if so for what aspects); a description of the etiquette of peer review; whether outside assessment of the statistics was being obtained; how much the referee should correct the English style; how much feedback the referee would get; how much the author would be told; how quickly his report was needed; and whether he would be paid for his services.

GUIDELINES

Some of Whimster's needs are covered in books (219,220) or by the guidelines suggested by the Council of Biology Editors (table XV) (10); other answers will depend on the journal's requirements. Nevertheless, several problems may still arise if the editor does not define the referee's role and focus his analysis.

A code prepared for the assessors to *Physics Today*, emphasized five aspects (221). Firstly, the referee has a central position and the journal's quality depends on the quality of his reviewing. Second, his task is to ensure that the article is as comprehensible as possible, so that his report

Table XV. Suggested guidelines for reviewers.

1. The unpublished manuscript is a privileged document. Please protect it from any form of exploitation. Reviewers are expected not to cite a manuscript or refer to the work it describes before it has been published, and to refrain from using the information it contains for the advancement of their own research.

2. A reviewer should consciously adopt a positive, impartial attitude toward the manuscript under review. Your position should be that of the author's ally, with the aim of promoting effective and accurate scientific communication.

3. If you believe that you cannot judge a given article impartially please return the manuscript immediately to the editor with that explanation.

4. Reviews should be completed expeditiously, within [state here the time you consider reasonable, for example, two weeks]. If you know that you cannot finish the review within the time specified, please telephone the editor (collect) to determine what action should be taken.

5. A reviewer should not discuss a paper with its author.

6. Please do not make any specific statement about the acceptability of a paper in your comments for transmission to the author, but advise the editor on this score either in a confidential covering letter with your comments or on the form(s) provided for that purpose.

7. In your review, please consider the following aspects of the manuscript as far as they are applicable:

    importance of the question or subject studied/originality of the work
    appropriateness of approach or experimental design/adequacy of experimental techniques
    soundness of conclusions and interpretation
    relevance of discussion
    clarity of writing and soundness of organization of the paper.

8. In comments intended for the author's eyes, criticism should be presented dispassionately, and abrasive remarks avoided.

9. Suggested revisions should be couched as such, and not expressed as conditions of acceptance. In a separate letter to the editor, please distinguish between revisions considered essential and those judged merely desirable.

10. Your criticisms, arguments, and suggestions concerning the paper will be most useful to the editor if they are carefully documented.

11. You are not requested to correct deficiencies of style or mistakes in grammar, but any help you can offer to the editor in this regard will be appreciated.

Table XV. (continued).

---

12. A reviewer's recommendations are gratefully received by the editor, but since editorial decisions are usually based on evaluations derived from several sources, a reviewer should not expect the editor to honour his every recommendation.

(Modified guidelines from the CBE (10), reproduced by its kind permission)

---

should be aimed at both the editor and the author. Third, because the sole contact is the written report, this must be both informative and explicit about the suggested action to be taken by the editor and what changes would make an article publishable. Fourth, a detailed report for the author is important and should concentrate on the manuscript's clarity. This should include three types of review: (*a*) a general impression about the important aspects; (*b*) a page by page notation of shortcomings or correction of logic, facts, and presentation, with close attention to the completeness of the data and pertinence of the tables and illustrations, and (*c*) an unambiguous list of required changes. Fifth, referees should not be caustic.

Dual publication
Some of the guidelines primarily aimed at authors may also help assessors. Thus the 'Relman-Ingelfinger rule' about previous publication emphasizes that the *New England Journal of Medicine* will consider manuscripts only with the understanding that neither the substance of the articles nor any of its illustrations or tables have been published or will be submitted for publication elsewhere (222). To a greater or lesser extent most other editors will go along with this, for dual publication is one of the most irritating and wasteful features of medical publishing today. Hence authors should state in their covering letter that the material has not been published previously or is currently being considered for publication elsewhere. Despite this, and a statement printed monthly, however, one editor found that three-quarters of the authors submitting articles still failed

to include an assurance about sole publication in their covering letter (223).

The guidelines issued by the International Committee of Medical Journal Editors distinguish between duplicate publication, which should not be allowed, and parallel publication—printing a different version of the article, usually in another language for a different readership with explicit reference to the primacy of the original publication (82)—which is permissible in certain circumstances.

Definition of an author

An author is someone who has taken a substantial part in both the study and writing of the article. The various statements about entitlement to be included as an author in an article include a statement by the Vancouver Group (224) and a clear explanation by Huth about who is entitled to be an author and who is not (table XVI) (217). The *Annals of Internal Medicine* now requires all authors of accepted articles to sign a condition of publication form, affirming that their names are on the paper in accordance with long-accepted criteria (225). Indeed, Burman has gone further than this, suggesting criteria for the order of the authors in an article and introducing the concept of the 'responsible author', who supervised the planning and execution of the study and the writing of the paper (226,227).

Ethics

Many sets of 'Instructions to Authors' remind them that their articles need to make explicit statements about the ethical aspects of a study. These should include whether informed consent and the approval of a hospital ethics committee were obtained and whether the protocol followed the procedure of the Helsinki Declaration for human or animal research (228).

Statistics

Altman has argued that a poor statistical basis for research is bad ethical practice and that ethics committees should

Table XVI. Criteria for authorship.

Basis for authorship Genesis of the paper	Legitimate	Not legitimate
Research report	Development of testable hypothesis	Suggestion that legitimate author(s) work on problem
Case report	First notice of previously unobserved phenomenon	Physician's, nurse's pharmacist's routine referral, care, service
Review	Critical inter-pretations of reviewed papers and assembled data	Suggestion that review be written
Research efforts	Study design Development of new method or critical modification of previous one	Suggestion of use of standard study design. Routine observations and measurements
Clinical studies	New diagnostic and therapeutic efforts	'Routine' diagnostic and therapeutic efforts
Interpretation	Explanatory insight into unexpected phenomena	Routine reports
Writing	First draft or critically important later revision	Solely criticisms of drafts and suggestions for revision of presentation
Responsibility for content	Ability to justify intellectually the conclusions of the paper	Solely attesting to accuracy of individual facts reported

(Reproduced from Hulk (217) by kind permission of the author and publisher)

automatically look at the experimental design of a study and the intended form of the analysis (229). It is fair to say, however, that many ethics committees would not agree with

Table XVII. Statistical guidelines for editors and referees.

---

1. Statisticians should help referees

2. All papers using any statistical procedure ought to be reviewed by a statistician

3. Revised papers should be returned to the same statistical referee for reappraisal

4. Journals using a statistical refereeing system should state clearly what their policy is

5. Journals should print statistical guidelines for contributors

6. Journals should encourage authors to supply additional information (especially on methods), which would help the referees but would not be for publication.

(Reproduced from Altman *et al.* (230) by their kind permission)

---

this and that they are not so constituted as to be able to practise his suggestions.

Few journals devote much of their 'Instructions to Authors' to statistics, and until recently editors and referees have also had little specific guidance. The guidelines by Altman and his colleagues apply equally well to authors, editors, or referees. Those for authors deal with requirements for the methods, results, presentation of results, and discussion and interpretation (230), and those for editors and referees have six main recommendations (table XVII).

In their reviewing, Altman *et al.* conclude, referees should ensure that there is adequate explanation and justification of what was done, while the conclusions must be reasonable and the abstract a fair reflection of the content. The referee's report should be understandable by authors who may have only minimal statistical training.

Almost twenty years ago statistical review for manuscripts submitted to *JAMA* was found to raise the proportion of statistically adequate papers published from 26 per cent of 514 studied before such review to 74 per cent of 161 published after this had been introduced. (Failure to reach 100 per cent statistical acceptability was said to be due to the editor's failing to resubmit all the revised papers to a

Table XVIII. Checklist for statistical review of papers for the
British Medical Journal.

BMJ Ref No: ——————   Date of Review: ——————

Design Features

1. Was the objective of the study sufficiently described?	Yes	Unclear	No
2. Was an appropriate study design used to achieve the objective?	Yes	Unclear	No
3. Was there a satisfactory statement given of source of subjects?	Yes	Unclear	No
4. Was there a power-based assessment of adequacy of sample size?	Yes	Unclear	No

Conduct of Study

5. Was a satisfactory response rate achieved?	Yes	Unclear	No

Analysis and Presentation

6. Was there a statement adequately describing or referencing all statistical procedures used?		Yes	No
7. Were the statistical analyses used appropriate?	Yes	Unclear	No
8. Was the presentation of statistical material satisfactory?		Yes	No
9. Were confidence limits given for the main results?		Yes	No
10. Was the conclusion drawn from the statistical analysis justified?	Yes	Unclear	No

Recommendation on Paper

11. Is the paper of acceptable statistical standard for publication?		Yes	No
12. If 'No' to Question 11, could it become acceptable with suitable revision?		Yes	No

Reviewer: ———————————————

(Reproduced from Gardner *et al.* (233) by their kind permission)

---

statistician.) The journal articles most needing such assessment tended to be those containing only a few probability
values and lacking statistical jargon (231).

Table XIX. *Checklist for statistical review of papers on clinical trials for the* British Medical Journal.

BMJ Ref No: _____   Date of Review: _____

Design Features

1. Was the objective of the trial sufficiently described?	Yes	Unclear	No
2. Was there a satisfactory statement given of diagnostic criteria for entry to trial?	Yes	Unclear	No
3. Was there a satisfactory statement given of source of subjects?	Yes	Unclear	No
4. Were concurrent controls used (as opposed to historical controls)?	Yes	Unclear	No
5. Were the treatments well defined?	Yes	Unclear	No
6. Was random allocation to treatment used?	Yes	Unclear	No
7. Was the method of randomization described?	Yes	Unclear	No
8. Was there an acceptable delay from allocation to commencement of treatment?	Yes	Unclear	No
9. Was the potential degree of blindness used?	Yes	Unclear	No
10. Was there a satisfactory statement of criteria for outcome measures?	Yes	Unclear	No
11. Were the outcome measures appropriate?	Yes	Unclear	No
12. Was there a power-based assessment of adequacy of sample size?	Yes	Unclear	No
13. Was the duration of post-treatment follow-up stated?	Yes	Unclear	No

Commencement of Trial

14. Were the treatment and control groups comparable in relevant measures?	Yes	Unclear	No
15. Were a high proportion of the subjects followed-up?	Yes	Unclear	No
16. Did a high proportion of subjects complete treatment?	Yes	Unclear	No
17. Were the drop-outs described by treatment/control groups?	Yes	Unclear	No

Table XIX. (continued).

BMJ Ref No: _____ Date of Review: _____

Design Features

18. Were side-effects of treatment reported?	Yes	Unclear	No

Analysis and Presentation

19. Was there a statement adequately describing or referencing all statistical procedures used?		Yes	No
20. Were the statistical analyses used appropriate?	Yes	Unclear	No
21. Were prognostic factors adequately considered?	Yes	Unclear	No
22. Was the presentation of statistical material satisfactory?		Yes	No
23. Were confidence limits given for the main results?		Yes	No
24. Was the conclusion drawn from the statistical analysis justified?	Yes	Unclear	No

Recommendation

25. Is the paper of acceptable statistical standard for publication?	Yes	No
26. If 'No' to Question 25, could it become acceptable with suitable revision?	Yes	No

Reviewer: _____

(Reproduced from Gardner *et al.* (233) by their kind permission)

A similar study for the *BMJ* confirmed the value of specific statistical reviewing, though it also emphasized how much assessors disagree about individual articles (232). As a result, our valued advisers, Gardner and his colleagues, introduced two checklists for use in peer review (tables XVIII and XIX) (233), and there are other similar guides (104,234,235).

Causation and cancer trials

Another useful checklist concerns the eight diagnostic tests for causation (table XX) (236), and a further one has recently been suggested for cancer trials (237).

Table XX. Diagnostic tests for causation.

1. Is there evidence from human experiments.
2. How strong is the association?
3. Do other investigators consistently find the same result?
4. Is there a gradient?
5. Does the association make epidemiological sense?
6. Does the association make biological sense?
7. Is the association specific?
8. Is the relationship analogous to another, well-accepted relationship?

(Reproduced from Sackett (236) by kind permission of the author and publishers.)

Such checklists can be applied to various aspects of the article and they are helpful to authors, editors, and assessors in reminding them of details that all of us tend to forget to consider. It is often a good thing for an editor to use them before he sends the article to a statistician, because then he can ask him specific questions about whether it is salvagable or not.

Therapeutic trials
A comparable approach may be used to study the reports of therapeutic trials (105). This checklist is in two parts: the first includes descriptions of the aim of the trial, the subjects, how the drugs or other therapeutic measures were used, and the experimental design and assessment; the second asks whether the criteria of a satisfactory therapeutic trial have been met, the data are adequately presented, and the conclusions are justified.

Untoward drug reactions
Similar criteria have been published for untoward drug reactions (106,238,239). All too often one reads manuscripts or even printed articles which lack sufficient details to enable the editor or reader to come to his own conclusions. The latest checklist for adverse drug reactions is that produced at the Morges Workshop. As previously

suggested, the minimal requirements are: age and sex of the patient(s), name and formulation of all drugs given; dosage of drug; duration of treatment; interval between starting treatment and appearance of the adverse drug reaction; and outcome of the adverse drug reaction—for example, complete or partial recovery (238).

An editorial in *Clinical Pharmacology* has urged authors to characterize adverse drug reactions as remote, possible, probable, or highly probable, and suggests that referees should consider two questions. Firstly, is the reaction well documented, either in the references or in primary publications? Second, is it 'ordinary'—for example, a minor skin reaction to a new antibiotic?

Forms for referees

In my survey (chapter 5) I found that about a quarter of the referees liked the forms I used and another tenth disliked them, in that both groups commented on them in separate letters. The former said that forms helped them to make up their minds and the latter said that they were too inflexible and inappropriate for experienced assessors. Nevertheless, forms may help the referees to crystallize their views and are useful for stating editorial policy on peer review—but referees should be free to use them or not (241). Such a suggestions is also supported by Cichetti, who found that reviewers agreed less when manuscripts were evaluated without the use of forms than with them (242).

Rating systems

A rating system for acceptability is advantageous, but there are no advantages in making it too complicated. An ambitious programme for two journals, *Murill-Palmer Quarterly* and *Developmental Review*, used a seven-point rating scale for 10 dimensions (74).[7] Those of us who like to keep things simple breathed a sigh of relief at the results: none of these was found to be a better indicator than a single 4-point summary judgment.

Part of this result is probably yet another example of a dissociation between what referees say about various aspects of an article and what they recommend (intersubjectivity, p. 66). Just as I found in my study that a colleague often tended to score all the criteria as 'moderate', and finally recommend acceptance, Cichetti also found that referees might class articles as having little scientific reliability or originality, and yet suggest that they should be accepted without change (242). So there is still a place for the editor to make his own judgments about reliability and validity (74), and there would be little sparkle to the job if there wasn't. Nevertheless, I believe that, if their limitations are accepted, checklists are valuable for all three members of the triangle (author, editor, and assessor): they can highlight errors of omission and commission, freeing everybody to concentrate on other aspects of the article—particularly the style and the logic.

Other possibilities

Similar checklists might also be feasible for other aspects of the article. For originality, for example, it might be possible to clarify this feature (table XXI:)

Another suitable item might be the references in the article. It is not unusual, for example, to find that accepted facts are documented by an absurd number of references— for example, 'cigarette smoking is associated with an increased incidence of cancer of the lung (1–20)' Such over-referencing was documented from a study of articles in the *Acta Medica Scandinavica*, which will now allow no more than 20 references per article (243,244).

NUMBER OF REFEREES

The number of assessors to be used in routine cases is often debated. At the *BMJ* we usually ask only one since statistically most articles are likely to be rejected; any that are considered suitable for publication after peer review are then read by the five medically qualified members of the hanging committee. At the other extreme, for *Current Anthropology* Belshaw argues strongly for 15 (ideally 20), chosen from various parts of the world, including the USSR,

Table XXI. Checklist for originality.

Unknown to me
Known to me:
  —unpublished (on grapevine)
  —presented at meeting (unpublished, published abstract, published
    paper in proceedings)
Published formally by same author already in part/whole
Closely/partly resembles similar work published by others

---

finding that 7–12 of these finally give an opinion (27).
This number, he says, is needed instead of the usual 1–3, to
counteract bias and to reveal differences of opinion, which
are particularly likely in this discipline; even then, possibly
only one out of 10 referees will comment on serious flaws in
the data, omissions in the references, and flawed methods.
In an editorial comment Harnad agrees that more than three
assessors are needed, but finds that *Behavioural and Brain
Sciences* can obtain a 100 per cent response from 5–8
assessors if they are contacted by telephone before being
sent the article (49,245).

I wonder about how rigorous the opinions are from so
many assessors, suspecting that if an individual referee
knows that his is one opinion among several he may tend to
be less than thorough. Probably, however, the ideal number
of assessors must be largely determined by the discipline,
and particularly by the degree that subjective factors,
including politics, are likely to influence judgments. In
Gordon's multidisciplinary survey (done in 1975), 23
journals used one 'critical external reader' per article, 11
two, and 1 three; four journals (the *Lancet*, the *Journal of
Medical Microbiology*, and two philosophy journals) used
none (36). Nevertheless, I suspect that today the commo-
nest practice is to use two external assessors, some editors
emphasizing that these should be deliberately chosen to
represent different standpoints, not only philosophically but
for their insights into the article (246). A young referee
may spend a lot of time going into the details of the work

(such as the experimental design, presentation, and analysis), while an older one will, though spending less time on the article, be better able to set it in the perspective of past findings and the implications of the work for the future (247). The difficulty about younger referees is that often they tend to put their report into the perspective of an ideal article rather than the inevitably imperfect one that they asked to comment on.

Blinding the referee to the author's identity is a possibility that authors raise more often than editors, some of whom already practise it (9,24,43,248). Indeed, one comment on the survey by Peters and Ceci is that the reader should assume that blind review is mandatory unless evidence to the contrary is forthcoming (248).

Blinding may be a partial remedy against bias in peer review: about two-thirds of the assessors for *Developmental Psychology* and *American Psychologist* cannot identify the authors (249). Questionnaires completed by two referees for each of 500 manuscripts submitted to the *American Journal of Public Health* showed that 279 pairs could not identify the author(s); in 109 cases both referees knew their identity and in 112 cases one referee knew and the other did not (Yankauer, personal communication). If neither referee knew who the author was, the consensus was greater than when they did, in which case they were more likely to recommend rejection. On the other hand, the degree to which authors are recognized may depend on the discipline: 80 per cent of authors of letters of *Physical Review Letters* can be identified by referees competent in the narrow subdiscipline (71).

Given that blinding is impossible to achieve all the time—the highest success rate being the 90 per cent for the *Canadian Medical Association Journal* (250)—Relman believes that the system is inequitable (38). One journal that offers the choice of blind review or not finds that very few authors opt for it (251). Nevertheless, I believe that the possibility of various biases and the suggestive evidence that these do sometimes operate (particularly giving rise to the Matthew effect) make blind reviewing a priority for consideration. In particular, I was struck by the theory (252,253) that referees make up their minds about an article in a minute or two (surely based on prejudices about the authors or subjects, or both) and then spend a couple of hours justifying their opinion—though how this could be verified is beyond me.

The difficulty over blind reviewing is that at present most articles abound with internal clues to the author's identities; merely detaching the first page of the text with their names and affiliations will not prevent referees from deducing who they are from phrases such as 'previous work from this laboratory (1–4)....' or the acknowledgements to identifiable colleagues or departments.

Authors, then, would need to style manuscripts for journals practising blind assessment specifically to exclude these clues, and one journal offers them this option to do this, with apparent success (26). Better still, a large journal should carry out a rigorous controlled trial of blind against open peer review, not forgetting that the editor, the editorial board, and the secretary responsible also all need to be blinded until a decision has been taken on the article. The protocol for such a study would be difficult, and the rigour for a valid answer would be a heavy burden on the editorial team—but the result would justify the cost.

SHOULD THE REFEREE SIGN?

The referee's role should be to criticize as an auxiliary, not as an adversary, Ingelfinger stated, maintaining that all reviews and comments to authors should be signed (116). In nine years as editor of the *New England Journal of Medicine* he had never seen an abrasive or insulting word used by a named reviewer, though signing did not imply emasculated opinions, any more than it did with editorials or book reviews. Ingelfinger pointed out that, though both of these had been anonymous, both were now usually signed; he predicted that by the end of the century signed assessors' reports would be the rule as well.

Another plea for signed referees' reports spoke of a sense of licence which anonymity confers to hand down opinions that are less than well documented. The strongly argued article, 'Towards open refereeing', maintained that to keep the assessor anonymous is almost as objectionable as his recommending rejection of an article without giving reasons (254). Open refereeing would enable authors to judge how competent a reviewer was, and would promote higher standards of peer review. Nevertheless, the article claimed, 'editors prefer anonymous refereeing because it is easier to run a journal where exchanges between authors and referees can be controlled and if need be subdued, not because it is necessarily science that benefits from such anonymity.'

Surely, however, this is taking the idea of conspiracy rather too far; the main reason for preserving anonymity is to avoid introducing more subjectivity into what should be as objective a practice as possible. The other side of the argument is as strongly put by Ziman, who denounces the call for disclosing the referees' names as 'populist folly' (255). Anonymity is better for all concerned: for the referee because he does not have to mix emotional factors with intellectual judgments; for the editor, who gets a more honest guide to his decisions; for the reader, who gets a more reliable and better expressed paper that has been subjected to a higher standard of criticism; and for the author, who when his mistakes are pointed out can vent his chagrin on an impersonal critic. And others have claimed that junior reviewers might hazard their promotion prospects if they were to criticize papers written by vindictive senior authors who also sit on appointment committees (249).

Just as important scientifically is the risk that signed review might not be critical enough to improve an article as much as it needs (250). We have no evidence that scientific objectivity would be preserved, and (just as named book reviewers seem to be more restrained than anonymous referees commenting on articles) referees might be tempted to write bland reports, which would have to be supplemented by their truthful opinions given to the editor on the telephone. Given all the evidence, therefore, I find it difficult to believe that a signed system would work in any smallish hierarchical society; my own feelings are 60:40 against it. A controlled study of this problem would be welcome but almost impossible to set up because it could never be truly random and too many confounding factors would be present.

One compromise would be to allow reviewers to sign if they wished: the *New England Journal of Medicine* (47) and the *Annals of Internal Medicine* (Huth, personal communication) have found that 15 per cent of assessors take this option. In January 1977 the *Journal of Laboratory and Clinical Medicine* encouraged their reviewers to sign their reports; in that year 68 per cent of reports recommending acceptance were signed compared with 59 per cent of those recommending rejection; in 1980 the respective figures were 60 per cent and 50 per cent (30). Seniority did not affect the decision to sign and the reports were by no means bland; letters to the editor about the practice were equally divided in their views. The editor comments that a pluralistic society has room for both views, and that he will continue to encourage reviewers to sign.

Another possibility would be to name referees either in a general list acknowledging their help over a year—a practice which several journals already follow—or by printing their name at the end of the articles (225,257). One belief is that this might pin some responsibility on the assessors in cases of piracy, plagiarism, or fraud. To my mind, however, it would abrogate editorial responsibility and give far too much apparent power to the referee.

EDITORS SHOULD EDIT!

At best a referee can make such a valuable contribution to a manuscript that arguably this deserves acknowledgement in the published paper. Again, however, most editors, would feel that this would place too much responsibility on the referees: ultimate decisions depend on all sorts of questions apart from those considered by a single referee—and often reflect style, taste, and so on (rather like wine tasting, as one contributor to the Peters and Ceci symposium comments (249)).

One of the more important of these, which I have no space to discuss, is economics. At the *BMJ* we accept papers of marginal quality depending on the current waiting list, but have never had to turn down papers that we would really liked to have accepted. Other journals, however, sometimes find that for reasons of cost they are declining as many as a fifth of the articles they would like to accept (Dudley, personal communication).

So editors should start to edit, declares Goodstein rather testily in the same symposium (258); do they actually read the articles themselves or are they merely clerks?[2]

In particular, their role is vital in deciding on the 'difficult' or 'absolutely wrong' articles (42), in adjudicating between referees, and in monitoring the latter, using the editorial board and their own knowledge and judgment for this (259); only in this way would we, for instance, know that, the more eminent the assessor, the more likely is he these days to refuse to referee an article or to give a poor opinion: for 1600 reports for the *Journal of Clinical Investigation* 74 per cent of 'low status' referees gave a good quality report compared with only 57 per cent of 'high status' ones (260).

Yalow, for example, also echoes the charges by others of incompetence (by both the editors and the reviewers) in the Peters and Ceci study (139). A Nobel prizewinner and a reviewer, when assessing a manuscript she always reads previous papers by the authors and also attempts to determine whether their work has been cited by others—routines which would have detected the Peters and Ceci deception straight away. This, of course, is one good argument against blinding the referee to the authors' identities.

Several commentators have argued that the editor should take up the referee's points with the author before he takes a final decision. Soffer, an opponent of signed reviews, considers such a dialogue essential, often with the aid of third or fourth reviewers (261). Another argument is that this dialogue ought to be between the authors and the reviewers directly (262), but surely a better alternative is for a similar but anonymous exchange to be carried out through the editor—who is still responsible for taking the final decision. And in fact this sort of exchange is what largely goes on already, for few articles are accepted without modification, and in many cases the decision depends on the reply to specific points or on the quality of additional data.

A further option with difficult articles is to publish them together with a commentary, possibly the unanswered comments of the referee printed at the end of the article (49). The journal that has gone the furthest in doing this is *Behavioural and Brain Research*, the one responsible for publishing the Peters and Ceci study. On the example of the 'participatory democracy' of some American Indian nations, it introduced the concept of open peer commentary (261). In this, signed comments are printed by the referees and other invited experts at the end of the article, together with a riposte by the author(s). This would seem an ideal way of dealing with the more difficult problem of the hypothesis-generating article rather than the hypothesis-confirming one. Many editors go half way with this, publishing an accompanying editorial with the article, allowing the authors to reply in a subsequent issue of the journal.

Publishing such commentaries might be easier if assessors listed the strengths of a manuscript as well as its weaknesses (262). I doubt, however, whether many editors would agree with yet another idea: that authors of a rejected manuscript should be able to choose whether to have a limited summary published in the journal. In this case they would have to deposit the complete text in a central agency, possibly together with a short but anonymous summary of the editor's reasons for rejection (124).

Finally, if editors are to accept Goodstein's challenge to start to edit they have to decide on their personal philosophy. Is their main role to record the minor but undoubted advances in their disciplines or to try to seize on the exciting but potentially wrong discovery and give it all the publicity they can? This question has been discussed in chapter 6.

SUMMING IT ALL UP: PERSONAL PREJUDICES

With so many suggestions and so few facts inevitably any summing up has to be based on yet another set of personal prejudices. To start with, I shall try to answer the questions asked earlier in this monograph. The first two, raised by Ingelfinger, are the most difficult to answer. To 'Is validation really secured by the conventional system of manuscript review?' the answer must be no: that is the role of time. We have seen that peer review has not detected fraud, plagiarism, or simple errors in, say, statistics—and, though an improved system might increase the likelihood of spotting the last two, it could not be expected to reveal fraud (unless, as in the case of mathematics, where referees test the equations by working them through, reviewers were to repeat the studies—clearly an impossibility).

Secondly, Ingelfinger asked whether peer review was worth the price. Though he posed this question in the context of a positive answer to the first, I believe that one answer may be given by replying to another: does peer review act as a filter or a traffic policeman, respectively preventing publication altogether or merely directing articles away from one journal to another? In my study I found, as did others, that some articles in the original sample remained unpublished. Possibly a few of these had been published elsewhere, and they could not be traced, or possibly, as Wilson found (39), their authors had been convinced by peer review that they were wrong. In any case, those articles that the *BMJ* did accept were considerably altered, usually because of suggestions by the referee— again, a finding confirmed by others.

Because of all this I believe that peer review is worth the price—which at £48 per article is small compared with the cost of the rest of a large journal's expenses (the current cost of a page of the *BMJ* is about £450). In any case, it is difficult to envisage going back to a system of in-house evaluation for, though a single journal might retain its reputation by using such a system, it is unlikely that all of them would get away with it—and even in-house refereeing is not cheap. Again, the scientific community has come to expect serious evaluation of submitted manuscripts and would not accept less. And my own study suggested that the combined contribution of editors screening articles, referees reading the remainder, and editors using the referees' opinions in making their final decision is as effective a mechanism as any for identifying those articles that should be published and then put to the test of time.

None of these conclusions are original but they are no less important or pressing for that. Firstly, despite all its faults, and the lack of overwhelming objective evidence for its value, editorial peer review, I believe, must remain in medicine and science: we have no better way of distinguishing between the promising and the meretricious or for improving the scientific and the linguistic qualities of an article. Apart from the evidence I have discussed in this book let me cite a recent will-o'-the-wisp idea that arose because of a lack of peer review. Pauling published his speculations on Vitamin C and Cancer in the *Proceedings of the National Academy of Science* (263). Usually this journal contains only peer reviewed articles, but members of the Academy have the right to publish an article without going through this process, which Pauling exercised, thereby exciting a considerable stir (263). And, on a more mundane level we may echo Soffer's questions: how many major studies published in the past fifty years have referred to articles in controlled circulation review journals or medical newspapers? (260).

Second, we must recognize the deficiencies of the system. Peer review does not, and cannot, ensure perfection: scientific journals are records of work done and not of revealed truth (264). If they were to insist on absurdly high standards science would suffer more than it would gain, purchasing reliability at the expense of innovative quality.

Some of these deficiencies are inherent; others can be eliminated or at least taken into account; yet others can be revealed by comments in subsequent Letters to the Editor, while there is always the role of time, for if the ideas are weighed in the balance and found wanting they will be discarded and ignored. Nevertheless, like all systems, peer review needs improving and we need rigorous research into both its process and outcome. Many of the changes discussed in this monograph would be feasible straight away, but to try to introduce them piecemeal would be a disaster, solving nothing.

Third, and finally, we have seen that science (including medicine) and peer review reflect each other's values; a fundamental improvement in peer review is likely to come about only when there has been a similar improvement in the attitudes of the scientific community, setting quality at a premium, and deriding rather than extolling spurious productivity.

The kind of research I envisage is discussed in Appendix I. Here, if we accept that peer review must stay, I shall conclude by discussing some of the improvements that are readily practicable.

If they cannot rely on a hanging committee to discuss articles every few weeks, then most editors will need to consult two assessors, and to diminish the Matthew effect I favour true blind reviewing, until I have been convinced that it is nugatory. The referees should be thought to be quick, competent, and fair, monitored frequently by the editor and a small editorial board. The latter should also ensure that referees are not overworked. Unless he wants to, no referee should be expected to review more than six articles in a year, given that each may well take him a day and that he will probably receive similar requests from other journals. If the two reviewers can be chosen for opposite attributes, so much the better, though this is not always possible. Choosing referees with a computer may overcome some of the editor's biases (265)—and it will enable him to select unknown ones as well as to monitor their performance.

Checklists are a help to many, but not all, referees, and editors should try to improve them as well as to develop fresh ones. Referees need to be told the eventual decision and to have a letter of explanation if it goes against their advice. They may be given the option of signing their reports if they want to. Separate statistical assessment (with the statistician told of any specific editorial queries as well as of the scientific referees' reports) should be sought for any suitable article that seems likely to be accepted.

Next an editor should reread the article in the light of the referee's report, deciding what is fair and what is not, and what changes are practicable and what are not, and he should censor any wounding phrases before sending the report to the author. Even if the article is rejected, however, the author is entitled to an explanation: the editorial and refereeing processes take an enormous amount of time, much of which will be wasted if these are viewed only as a sorting and not also as an educational exercise. Conversely the author must accept that not all rejections are based on scientific doubts about the article, but may reflect the editor's taste and judgment (which if he is a good editor will be as wide and generous as possible).

Finally, all editors should aim at some sort of continual audit of their practices; how many times do they use a referee a year, what is the quality of his reports, and is he or she demonstrably wrong, biased, or slipshod? They should also try to follow subsequent judgments on the articles that pass through their hands both published and rejected but published elsewhere.

Such research may sound a tall order, particularly for a part-time editor with little help—though it should become easier with a computer and the use of citation analysis (particularly the newer refined measurements, such as weighting factors[3] (20)), but I believe that it is essential. Publication occupies such a key position in science that it is extraordinary that no one, inside or outside the editorial office, has studied it in the depth that its importance demands.

So, in ending with the question as to who is right (p.

21), I finish by supporting Ziman that peer review is the lynchpin of science (46), though I have a sneaking suspicion that all too often Sir Theodore Fox has the last laugh (3).

APPENDIX I

Priorities for action

I believe that the need for action to study and improve peer review is pressing. Most commentators on the information explosion have written as if they were the first to confront it, ignoring similar talk about a crisis years beforehand. Both Bernal in 1939 and Fox in 1963 made similar proposals for stemming the flood of new journals—establishing two different types of journal (the newspaper and the archival)—but nothing happened save the flood is now even more apparent (26). But, at the risk of seeming another Jeremiah to be proved wrong in a further generation, I believe that today serious new stresses and strains have been added to these problems: the static or declining funding for research, a consistent annual fall of 3–5 per cent in the circulation of most learned scientific journals (266), and the impact of the new technology (though this might help to solve the problems as well).

THE NEW TECHNOLOGY: FANTASY

Several fantasies have been published about the impact of the last of these. My own, 'Brave New Journals: 2033', envisages that a crisis occurred in the year 2000 caused by the ever-increasing number of articles, mostly of poor quality, and the plague of shady practices—particularly piracy, plagiarism, and forgery (267). Added to this, governments had forbidden drug advertisements because, they alleged, these had influenced doctors to prescribe expensive drugs wrongly, while journals had lost their advertisements for job vacancies to Teletext, obtainable by anybody on his own domestic television set.

By 1995, then, the yearly subscription to a weekly

medical journal had run to $1000, and most doctors had cancelled their subscriptions. The solution to the crisis caused by a lack of communication, together with the necessary subsidies, had come from the World Health Organization: one general journal and one set of specialist journals for each of the principal medical zones of the world (Europe, Australasia, America, and Asia), all published in English in a uniform format and style.

The mass of publications had been severely reduced by several measures. Firstly, when starting research all investigators registered their projects with a central data bank; this ensured that nobody unwittingly duplicated research (though it did not prevent their embarking on confirmatory or refutatory work). Second, any applicant for a post could submit only six published papers as a testimony to his work—hence the emphasis was on its quality with an abolition of the pressure on journals to publish 'salami' articles about work in progress. Third, most reports of drug side-effects and negative results (which were still peer reviewed) were stored in a computer databank. Fourth, during registration at the journal all new articles were fed into another databank to see whether they had been published elsewhere or were being considered for publication.

Finally, in this fantasy, articles would be transmitted between the author, editor, and referee by telephone line on to a word-processor; referees would be chosen by computer; and standard codes had been devised, and their use insisted on, for basic medical English, statistics, and authorship. Peer review was blind, though the assessors signed their reports. As a result of all this, many major men and women in medicine now wrote only two or three articles in their lives—their other communications being with the invisible colleges, particularly at workshops, which had replaced large and useless international medical jamborees.

THE NEW TECHNOLOGY: REALITY

Whatever the fantasies, clearly almost immediately the new technology may help to solve some economic problems, particularly of those scientific journals with small circulations and of the new ones that will be started to cross the disciplines whatever the complaints that there are too many already. For some years law reports have been available in a database for retrieval in the office or home, and in 1984–5 four general medical journals (*Annals of Internal Medicine, British Medical Journal, Lancet, and New England Journal of Medicine*) also went on line; this system is now being rapidly expanded to take in the specialist archival journals (268,269).

With this database each individual page of the journal can be retrieved, apart from complex tables and illustrations. These should be transmittable soon, and most of us welcome such developments. The dissemination of knowledge should be faster and more comprehensive; unchecked photostating (a threat to the survival of some publications) should be discouraged; and, compared with the conventional media, it should be cheaper—though, to offset this, it may diminish the sales of hard copies to present day subscribers.

Database retrieval is, however, merely publication in another, and supplementary, form and many journals will always be produced in the conventional archival form after peer review. The new proposals for totally electronic journals pose much larger problems, particularly for peer review.

Those journals envisaged by the Comtec Corporation would have disseminated material quickly after peer review (usually rapid and internal), paying the author $100 for each article published. The major source of material would have been the progress reports scientists have to file periodically with the granting agencies funding the research (270).

Plotkin's keynote address about these plans to the annual meeting of the Council of Biology Editors in 1982 provoked a stormy discussion, in which the validity of the peer review and the enshrinement of the electronic text as an archive figured prominently (271). Electronic developments are inevitable, however, and it is important to anticipate such problems as we can, using our experience of conventional publication and instituting an audit of the effects of the new technology.

In the past year, moreover, other similar plans have come to fruition (269). *Clinical Notes On-Line* is published both electronically and conventionally as a printed monthly journal (272). It aims at harvesting 'the vast body of interesting, unique, and unusual cases that all doctors encounter from time to time'. Using a standard format, authors can submit brief contributions by post, or 'upload' them by telephone from their own microcomputers to the journal office. Electronic handling may also be used for peer review and correspondence with the author and should ensure prompt publication: provided the editor does not have to refer back to the author, contributions will be included in the *CNOL* database within an average of three weeks of receipt.

Against the advantages of speed, priority, and low-cost have to be set the risks of inaccuracy, duplication, and triviality. True, the *CNOL* editors do scrutinize articles, and the databases and printed versions may include their comments and subsequent ones—yet its policy statement maintains that 'communications must be regarded as original, unreviewed observations' and it continues by emphasizing that '*the authors* accept professional responsibility for their reports' (my italics). Similar objections were raised in 1973 to the rapid publication *Journal of International Communication Research Studies*, which prints reports within five to six weeks of receipt (273). Defending this, Horrobin claimed that the journal was only formalizing the current invisible colleges (274). Quality control was ensured by emphasizing objective criteria such as the number of patients or experiments and the presence or absence of statistical treatment.

Much the same doubt must be expressed about suggestions that doctors might input, say, single instances of adverse drug reactions into a database by themselves without peer review. There are also bound to be doubts about 'interactive' reports, which in the database may be changed by the original author, the reviewer, or the reader (though it is stated that the text of each version will remain accessible in the archive). Who is to validate such reports, ensuring that these will not produce false fears or reassurances, even if standardized formats are used? Any non-specialist who has seen the print-out of 'drug side effects,' produced by the Committee on the Safety of Medicines, will know how confusing the mass of such sporadic and apparently contradictory reports may be, even though in this case they have been rigorously filtered for quality.

Finally, it should not be forgotten that conventional publication still has advantages over the electronic form. In 1982 de Solla Price's first paper was cited for the first time. He had published this in 1946 in the *Mathematical Gazette*, but at that time did not belong to any invisible college and his work was ignored. Nevertheless, the full text went into the archives, whence it was retrieved 36 years later; until this is possible with the new medium, Price believed that the conventional form was preferable (142).

RESEARCH INTO PEER REVIEW

Calls for research into peer review go back some years, almost all of them, however, exhortations rather than detailed proposals. One of the latter is an unpublished project for a four-year study of the life history of manuscripts submitted to biomedical or biology journals in the USA, and it is worth using this in discussing some principles and practices.

This project was to study four aspects of peer review: its impact on the course, content, and fate of the manuscript; its cost; the editors' reasons for their individual decisions; and data about the system's effectiveness. Of the three stages of the study, the first would list all institutions and agencies recording articles and reports sent for publication (such as the two discussed by Roland and Kirkpatrick and Mundy (12,78)), and take a sample. Second, a medical discipline would be chosen, and a sample of departmental chairmen asked to rank the relevant journals in order of prestige. Each of these would then be asked about the following: the number of manuscripts received and published; the system of screening and peer review; the turnround time to publication; editorial decision-making; and a list of regular reviewers.

The third and final stage would study a sample of papers sent to a sample of journals (say, 10), with the survey staff correlating data on these. The authors would be asked about the past history of the manuscript, for a copy of both the initial and any revised versions, and for their reactions to the reviewers' and editors' comments. The editors would be asked for the assessors' comments and the reasons for their decisions. The referees would be asked how many hours they had spent on a manuscript, while finally there would be a retrospective study of papers published by all the journals in the discipline under study.

COMMENTS

Sample size

As the document emphasizes, these proposals were tentative. Many details remained to be worked out, depending on the reaction of those approached and the findings of a pilot trial. Nevertheless, as one of the few proposals ever put on paper, it is worth commenting on its details as well as its principles, and I can do so as one whose own study was less than comprehensive. Firstly, then, I suspect that the samples, both of the journals and of the articles, were too small to give meaningful results.

Co-operation

Second, the proposals were optimistic about co-operation from the various participants. In my study it took an inordinate amount of work to obtain an 80 per cent response rate to my questionnaire from the authors; many assessors, I suspect, would not be willing for their reports to be released outside the privileged circle of editor and author; and I can think of one or two editors or their publishers who will not co-operate with anybody.

National orientation

A third criticism would be that the project was entirely American orientated; if the subdiscipline studied were, say, cardiology, it might seriously distort any findings if the British, European, or Scandinavian journals on cardiology or hypertension were ignored. Hence any research project must be truly international.

Quality

Fourth, though the proposals were strong on process, they failed to address one vital feature of outcome: quality. There was no mention of its assessment by citation analysis or consensus analysis by experts, as has been done for schistosomiasis (160) or hepatitis (162).

Emphasis

To go on with comments and suggestions would be to pillory a proposal that might have been utterly changed in its definitive form, reflecting many of these points. My final comment, however, would be that, to obtain the co-operation of at least two members of the triangle, *any* study should be author-centred rather than editor-centred (and I suspect that the referee would be more interested in this emphasis as well). To be sure, editors are fascinated by what happens to articles they reject, but authors and reviewers would like answers to more immediate questions. Is peer review 'fair'? Would it be fairer with two reviewers rather than one, three rather than two, and so on. What would be the real impact of blinding the referee to the authors' identities? Given limited resources, would a formal appeal mechanism be cost-effective for all concerned?

That these are some of the questions to be answered also emerges from the recent suggestions by Bailar and Patterson, who call for a thorough analysis of journal peer review policy and relevant research needs (121). Other possible investigations, they suggest, include: seeing whether more manuscripts could be assessed without external review; investigating the filter and the traffic policeman functions of peer review by tracking a set of manuscripts; comparing the efficacy of different sets of 'Instructions to Authors'; and evaluating the nature, extent, costs, and impact of changes suggested by reviewers.

THOROUGH ANALYSIS

It is time, Bailar and Patterson conclude, to recognize that peer review is an important object of study which may improve the use of journals to promote scientific advances. Some group or agency should now undertake the necessary thorough analysis. Half a dozen senior investigators, with some supporting staff but little else in the way of resources, could make substantial progress on most critical issues.

I support their proposal, even though they underestimate the task and the demands it will make, and even though an office joke is the stereotyped final phrase in articles, whether commissioned editorials or submitted original work: 'more research is needed'. Such research will not be easy and it is vital to get the methods defined and agreed, both nationally and internationally. Even when money is as short as it is today, there is a strong case, I believe, for the three main bodies concerned—the universities, granting agencies, and journals—to get together and plan and finance such a project. To any one organization the cost would be small, but the potential savings are immense.

Such a large-scale research programme should be sponsored by a disinterested major national or international body. This sponsorship might also make it easier to change our current attitudes, by shifting the scientific community's preoccupation with quantity to one with quality, especially in making its status judgments. In particular, can we develop and use better criteria for quality without impeding important advances or threatening the openness of science?

In answering all these questions cross disciplinary studies may give the most valuable answers. Why, for instance, are there such differences among the disciplines and yet overall the end results seem much the same?

In any scientific discipline about 80 per cent of the

articles written get published. One discipline has recognized this. Its journals have grown out of all proportion to the increase in the number of scientists working in it and the first journal approached can publish most of the articles it receives (though usually after changes resulting from rigorous peer review) (71). Another discipline has not recognized that peer review acts principally as a traffic policeman, or its philosophy is that the subject is better 'split' than 'lumped' (to mix my metaphors again), or there is a mixture of both attitudes. Hence editors and referees work hard to achieve a high initial rejection rate; others successively do the same so that these rejected articles are sped through other journals down an ever-steeper slope of esteem.

Are both of these practices right, determined by the needs of the discipline? In physics, an example of the 'tolerant' discipline, where a few journals act as a sponge, a relaxed attitude to publication may do little ultimate harm, even though it is here that only 15 per cent of articles contain useful information (157). In medicine, where peer review acts as a traffic policeman, do the high rejection rates reflect fears that flawed work might harm patients or provoke public alarm—and if either of these is true, why do the editors of general and specialist medical journals have such different criteria? Could the final rejection rates be higher in all disciplines (say, 40 per cent of all articles remaining unpublished) with the traditional openness of science still preserved, and what could one discipline learn from another? The differences among them need exploring—for example, why citation practices vary so much. Mathematicians cite less than half as many papers as biochemists; engineers, on the other hand, cite books as heavily as journals, as do the social scientists (275).

Finally, can we really say that all of these articles (in whatever subject) are 'necessary', given that from the outset many of them are known to be flawed and subsequently are never referred to at all? These are the questions,[1] but what are the answers?

APPENDIX II

Semantics

The terminology of peer review generates a surprising amount of interest and emotion. Indeed, is 'peer review' the right term for the process, given the alternatives of 'refereeing' or 'assessment for publication'? Is 'peer reviewer' right for the person who does it, given the alternatives of 'referee, assessor, consultant, or adviser'?

The one official pronouncement on semantics was in 1981 at the second assembly of the International Federation of Scientific Editors Associations. This distinguished between reviewing and refereeing: the former should be limited to judgments made *after* publication (such as book reviews); and the latter should be used for a quality judgment made *before* publication (277). Nevertheless, few attempts have been made to follow these recommendations, even by the members of IFSEA, so that next we must turn to the dictionaries. These help over definitions and dates (278) but not in distinguishing the merits of the alternatives. Thus the origins of referee go back to:

(1456) *Refer*. To commit, submit, hand over (a question, cause, or matter) to some special or ultimate authority for consideration, decision, execution etc.

(1670) *Referee*. One to whom any matter or question in dispute is referred for decision; an umpire.

(1884) *Referee*. A person appointed to examine a scientific or other learned work and comment on its suitability for publication.

(1649) *Review*. A general account or criticism of a literary work.

The *Oxford English Dictionary* also shows that in Britain 'peer'—an equal in civil standing or rank—goes back to 1215, with a mention in Latin in *Magna Carta* (and in France even earlier, with Charlemagne's douzepers or

Rerences begin on p. 164

paladins). The more recent anthropological and social usage is of an equal; a contemporary; a member of the same age group or social set. Under this heading the *Supplement* to the *Oxford English Dictionary* quotes *Nature* (1975): 'At the heart of the inquiry is the so-called peer-review system, which is used in some shape or form by virtually every government agency which supports academic research' (279).

Clearly these terms for the same activity might have opposite meanings: one of the definitions of referee, an umpire, is derived from *non per*, an unequal. But this is to burden the expert assessor with an unnecessary load. His role is not as an umpire or referee in the sense of adjudicating between two diametrically opposed sides: he is there as one of the editor's sources of expert advice on an article's merits, not for making the final decision whether to accept the paper, with or without revision, or to reject it for publication.

Both terms have their difficulties when it comes to derivations; to 'peer review' sounds odd as a verb and there is no noun corresponding to the verb 'to referee' to denote the subject, discipline, or profession of the referee, other than the awkward gerund 'refereeing'.

As a basis for making up my own mind I sent a questionnaire asking about their use and understanding of the terms 'refereeing' and 'peer review', with any comments, to a small group of editors, assessors, and lexicographers drawn from countries all over the world. Though fascinating, their replies gave little consensus to guide me about what was done and what should be done.

Thus, of the 38 questionnaires returned (table XXII), 17 considered that refereeing was the same as peer review, 19 did not, and two said that they were not quite the same thing (table). In distinguishing between the two, most people fell back on a literal definition of peer, pointing out that this implied that the assessor was of equal status to the author, whereas he was usually an authoritative expert with knowledge far superior to that of most authors.

One respondent suggested that peer review was done by

Table XXII. Use of 'peer review' or 'refereeing' by editors of medical journals and others.

	No
Editors replying to questionnaire	38
Theoretical discrimination of terms	
They are the same thing	17
They are not the same thing	19
They are not quite the same thing	2
Use of terms in practice	
Peer review	9
Refereeing	22
Either	4
Neither[1]	3
Additional comments supplied	
Referee is the arbiter when peer reviewers disagree	2
Peer review is for grants, referee for journal articles	2
Peer review is by equals, refereeing by expert	9
Peer review is for general journals, referee for specialist	1
Dissertations on etymology	2
Anti-American abuse of peer review[2]	4
Anti-sport abuse on refereeing[3]	4

1. Used 'independent assessment', 'professional co-workers', or simply 'review'.
2. Such as 'an appalling Americanism suggesting Nosey Parker and Big Brother', 'pandering to American Newspeak'.
3. 'Gladiator connotation'.

an author's associates before he submitted it for publication to the journal, which then refereed it; another considered that reviewing was a grander concept than refereeing, the terms being applied respectively to grant applications and job promotions or submitted articles; another thought that refereeing was done by the editorial board after peer review of the article by outside assessors; and yet another indicated that peer review could be applied to an assessment of an article by an expert working in the same discipline, but that refereeing was the right term if the opinion of an adviser outside the discipline was sought, such as that of a statistician. One editor thought that the processes were different for general journals or specialist journals: for the former the editor wanted the opinion of a generalist (peer reviewer), for the latter an expert authority (referee).

Finally, the confusion that may exist about terminology, even among colleagues, was shown by the widely diverse replies of 17 members from the office of a single large general journal. If none of the staff here are talking about the same thing, what hope is there for the rest of us?

OTHER COUNTRIES, OTHER WORDS

For good measure, to add to the confusion, some editors of journals published in languages other than English told me of the terms used in their countries; in French, referee may be translated into 'censeur', with its strong connotation of court martial (at least, so my informant told me), or, at the other extreme, 'lecteur', sounding warm and ambiguous; the Germans use Kritik and Italians critico; directly translated, the Norwegian term, 'faglige medarbeidere' means professional co-workers, while the Danes may use 'konsultant'. Any country, apparently, may just use the English word referee itself.

One of the more frequent comments made by the English editors was that peer review was American jargon ('an appalling Americanism suggesting Nosey Parker and Big Brother—designed to see whether doctors are doing their work properly') and its use in Britain 'pandering to American Newspeak'.

I always regret the supposition that only the English are the rightful guardians of the language and that the colourful and useful words and phrases originating in the USA should be treated with suspicion until they have been weighed in some traditional balance and found acceptable. Such a tradition goes back a long way: elected an honorary member of the American Academy, Thomas Jefferson wrote from Monticello on 21 January 1821 (280);

There are so many differences between us and England, of soil, climate, culture, productions, laws, religion and government, that we must be left far behind the march of circumstances were we to hold ourselves rigorously to their standards... Judicious neology can alone give strength and copiousness to language and enable it to be the vehicle of new ideas.

Nor can one fall back on the literal meaning of a word to damn its everyday usage in a context that everybody understands; one has only to cite the word tory—which originally meant an outlaw, being applied in the seventeenth century to the disposessed Irish, who kept alive by plundering the English settlers and soldiers. Today, after all, the word peer is 'applied loosely to any member of a group, without implying equality, and there is nothing wrong with Vercueil's definition of peer review: 'a term which may be applied to any system in which a group whose members are broadly equal in terms of status and qualifications chooses a panel from amongst its members to assess critically the activities of individuals in that group for some specific purpose' (281).

DECISIONS, DECISIONS

Hence I had to make up my own mind about what terms to use, choosing 'peer review' for the process and 'referee, assessor, reviewer, consultant, or adviser' for the person who carried it out. Here I have used the former as the general term for the assessment not only of articles for publication but also of grant applications, of a doctor's handling of his clinical responsibilities, or of the performance of a medical faculty. (I have not discussed the last two of these, though interestingly this type of peer review was what laymen immediately thought I was writing about when I mentioned my project.) The nouns I have used interchangeably as meaning the same.

The arguments on terminology were balanced, it seemed to me, but I was swayed in my decision by an opinion by Dr

Appendix II: Semantics

Edward J. Huth, editor of the *Annals of Internal Medicine* and the longest-serving editor of a major general medical journal in the world. Let him have the last word.

'I very much prefer,' Huth wrote, '"peer review" to "refereeing." "Refereeing" implies to me an unequivocal decision as to "right" or "wrong", or "out of the game" or "still in the game". There are certainly many papers of which one can say there are "right" or "wrong" but in clinical journals, it seems to me, we more frquently deal with "more likely to be right" and "more likely to be wrong". Many other factors influence our decisions as to what to accept, and the referee's verdict of "out of the game" or "still in the game" is not enough for many editorial decisions. I confine my use of "refereeing" to a function I assign to members of my editorial board, namely, rendering of a third critical opinion when two "peer reviewers" show strong disagreement. We prefer to refer to our "peer reviewers" as "consultants", a usage that carries the connotation that the ultimate editorial decision is up to us and that it is based only in part on the critical opinions of those whom we have consulted about particular papers'.

NOTES

CHAPTER 4

[1] One obvious comment would be the usual one whenever citation analysis is discussed. Nobody can be certain how much of this difference is due to quality and how much to the journal of publication—in other words, would the citation patterns have been partly reversed if the rejected articles had been published in the *JCI* and the accepted ones elsewhere? This is another illustration of our search for a gold standard for articles and the difficulties of having to rely almost entirely on citation analysis.

[2] The Uniform Requirements for Manuscripts Submitted to Biomedical Journals (82) suggest adding Abstract in brackets after the reference.

[3] These were: the absence of a control group when this was necessary; the absence of measures of sensitivity or specificity in evaluating a treatment, drug, or diagnostic procedure; improper use of statistical techniques; improper conclusions after proper statistical tests; inappropriate design of a study for solving a problem; no use of statistical tests when these were needed; use of the probability calculated on a given test as the true probability when many statistical tests had been applied to the same data; small power of the study; statement about significant differences without any description of the test used or the level of significance; conclusions drawn about a population but no test on sample to see whether these were justified (the most frequent error); misleading tables or charts; and improper manipulation of data.

CHAPTER 5

[1] This figure is 707 instead of 726 because in 19 cases the external reviewer was one of the consultants sitting on the hanging committee who was used for his expert knowledge.

CHAPTER 6

[1] It was, after all, the failure by distinguished American physicists to continue publishing regularly during the second world war that led a Soviet physicist to deduce that the USA was constructing an atomic bomb—a remarkable instance of Kremlinology in reverse.

[2] Just as important is the publicity given to any report of an

investigation showing no evidence of scientific fraud—as, for example, that of the inquiry vindicating the follow-up study by the Sobells of alcoholics practising controlled drinking (133).

³ This need for infallibility is something the editors of special journals share with the selection of Nobel laureates and the canonization of saints. When the validity of a scientific contribution is in doubt, the judges reject it in favour of a more securely based one, and the procedure for canonization has been formalized and restricted to rule out erroneous selection (54).

⁴ Sir Theodore Fox was a past master at this but examples of his interventions are not documented. So I will quote instead Thomas Park's letter to Lindeman about his trophic-dynamic theory in ecology, in which he acted against the advice of two eminent assessors. 'I have carefully considered your reviewed manuscript and am herewith accepting it for *Ecology*. I rather imagine that the original referees will still object to certain of its basic premises, but I think it best to publish your paper regardless. Time is a great solace in these matters and it alone will judge the questions' (136).

⁵ There are also a few isolated reports of prejudice in the other direction. 'A distinguished physicist once remarked in jest that nobody believed Wegener [who after some years was accepted as being right] because he obviously had a bee in his bonnet about Continental Drift, whereas Jeffreys [who had calculated that the theory was impossible], a shy and retiring man, obviously had nothing to gain or lose by it!' (46). An eminent pathologist stated that the Rous sarcoma could not be a cancer since Rous had discovered its cause (54).

⁶ Should anybody cite Mendel, it has to be pointed out that his work was published in a mainstream journal, copies of which found their way promptly to the major science libraries; what is surprising is that the biological community then took little notice of it for many years, probably partially because of its resistance to mathematics (137).

⁷ If there is such an entity as an operatic paradigm shift then it would apply to the operas composed by Leos Janáček: 'there are few operatic vocabularies which abandon the claims of music's own logic so extensively' (145). If, moreover, professional critics can help the non-expert by explaining these difficulties, their abilities should be tested to the full by *Osud* (*Fate*): a difficult work to stage, on the surface its plot is barely credible, and it was the last of Janáček's major operas to be performed.

While I was planning this monograph its first stage production in Britain took place at the English National Opera (September 1984), and through the kindness of its press office I obtained the major reviews and compared the performance of the music critics. One critic found the libretto convincing, another unconvincing; one who considered that the libretto was naive because it had been entrusted to a young woman was contradicted by another who pointed out that she had followed the composer's precisely stipulated needs.

For two critics the translation was strong and clear, for one it left him unable to catch the words. The production was variously described as a triumph of staging, brilliant, a brilliant solution to the problems, uncomprehending, and not meeting the al fresco needs. For three critics the orchestra was tentative, needing more time for rehearsal, or had yet to meet the conductor's passion; for two it swept all before it or caught the opera's spirit. Finally, a lengthy analysis in the *Times Literary Supplement* alone pointed to numerous instances where the composer's requirements had not been met (including the 'potted palm' in the couple's living room in the second act, intended as a wry comment on their marriage) and argued that the opera had yet to be staged.

Hence I would support the American painter Barnet Newman's adage that art criticism and theory are as much use to artists as onithology is to birds. The lack of critical consensus among music critics hardly supports Ruderfer's call for professional scientific referees.

[8] In fact, in 1984 it weighed 37kg and occupied 14 volumes.

[9] To see whether filtration by consensus might help readers an experiment was conducted a few years ago to review the publications on viral hepatitis. In the English language serials in the Medline file over 10 years ago there were no fewer than 16,000 citations. Nevertheless, by using 40 recent reviews on the subject a knowledge base of only 575 original articles was constructed. When a panel of 10 experts was asked to update this base they were confronted with another 5700 new articles published in the previous two and a half years—clearly an impossible load for any individual to come to grips with.

The solution was to look at which journals had published the initial 575 articles: 47 per cent of these had appeared in only five journals, and 80 per cent in 18 journals (among which, I was glad to see, was the *BMJ*). By using only the 18 journals, therefore, the experts were able to update the knowledge base and to arrive at a final number of only 620 articles.

CHAPTER 7

[1] The National Institutes of Health already use a review system involving laymen. Intially the proposals are studied by one of the 50 sections composed entirely of non-governmental scientists. Their recommendations go to an advisory council composed of non-governmental scientists together with laymen. This system is said to combine the intrinsic criteria of scientists (presumably newness, trueness, and scientific importance) with the extrinsic criteria of government agencies (presumably practical importance) (195).

[2] Taking past research performance into account in distributing funds has now been tried at Imperial College, London, which uses a complex formula, including the number of publications (but not citation analysis), the awards of prizes and medals, and elections to Fellowships

of the Royal Society and to senior positions in professional organizations (189).

[3] *Confidentiality over peer review.* Lest it be thought that peer review is not now considered to play a valuable part in assessing applications for research fundings, the opposite and traditional view has been supported by the US Courts (210). The Dow company tried to obtain the data on a long-term federally funded study of the effects of dioxin on rhesus monkeys, but a district court ruled that the disclosure of data to a company with vested interests could jeopardize a costly study and that the public interest was better served by witholding data until after peer review.

CHAPTER 8

[1] These were overall quality; impact, as measured by citations or controversy; conceptualization of problem; importance; importance of topic; originality of treatment; quality of writing; theoreticality; reliability of results; validity of conclusions; and breadth of interested audience.

[2] I would echo this comment; a very few editors of specialist journals (not those published by the BMA) send literally every article to two referees, reject if both advise this, referee if the two disagree, and read it only if two recommend acceptance. Such a practice is not editing, but could (almost) be done by a computer—and probably will be.

[3] Some journals receive more citations than they give out to other journals; the first divided by the second is known as the influence weight. If this is multiplied by the number of references per publication it yields the influence per publications, so compensating for editorial policies which might affect the number of references in an article. Thus a review journal containing only lengthy review articles will have a reference per publication value of 6–10 times that of a research journal, and so a large influence per publication (20). It remains to be seen how useful these two and other weighting factors will prove to be in practice, and whether they will refine the present criteria used in ordinary citation analysis.

APPENDIX I

[1] Just before [Gertrude Stein] died she asked, 'What is the answer?' No answer came. She laughed and said 'In that case, what is the question?' (276).

REFERENCES

1   Strutt RJ. *The Life of Lord Rayleigh.* London: Edward Arnold, 1924.

2   Ingelfinger RJK. Peer review in biomedical publication. *Am J Med* 1974;56:686–92.

3   Fox TF. *Crisis in communication.* London: Athlone Press, 1965.

4   Tocqueville AHCMC de. *De la democratie en Amerique.* Paris, 1835.

5   Zuckerman H, Merton RK. Patterns of evaluation in science: institutionalisation, structure and functions of the refereeing system. *Minerva* 1971;9:66–100.

6   Booth CC. Medical communication: old and new. Development of medical journals in Britain. *Br Med J* 1982;285:105–8.

7   Wilson JD. The Journal of Clinical Investigation 1974. *J Clin Invest* 1974;54: xv–xvii.

8   Relman AS. Moscow in January. *N Engl J Med* 1980;302:532–4.

9   Crane D. The gatekeepers of science: some factors affecting the selections of articles for scientific journals. *American Sociologist* 1967;2:195–201.

10 De Bakey L. *The scientific journal: editorial policies and practices.* St Louis: Mosby, 1976.

11 Koshland DE. An editor's quest.2. *Science* 1985;227:249.

12 Roland CG, Kirkpatrick RA. Time lapse between hypothesis and publication in the medical sciences. *N Engl J Med* 1975;292:1273–6.

13 Ingelfinger FJ. The general medical journal: for readers or repositories? *N Engl J Med* 1977;296:1258–64.

14 Woolf P. The second messenger: informal communication in cyclic AMP research. *Minerva* 1975;13:349–73.

15 Price D de S. The development and structure of the biomedical literature. In: Warren KS, ed. *Coping with the biomedical literature.* New York: Praeger, 1981;3–16.

16 Garvey WD. *Communication: the essence of science.* Oxford: Pergamon Press, 1979.

17 Carson J, Wyatt HV. Delays in the literature of medical microbiology: before and after publication. *Journal of Documentation* 1983;39:155–65.

18 Carson J, Wyatt HV. Retrieving references on microbiology: which secondary publications can help? *ASM News* 1982;48:5–9.

References

19   Moravcsik MJ. Rejecting published work: it couldn't happen in physics! (or could it?). *Behavioral and Brain Sciences* 1982;5:228–9.

20   Narin F, Pinski G, Gee HF. Structure of the biomedical literature. *Journal of the American Society for Information Science* 1976;January/February:24–45.

21   Garfield E. Citation analysis as a tool in journal evaluation. *Science* 1972;178:471–9.

22   Carter GM. *Peer review, citations, and biomedical research policy: NIH grants to medical school faculty.* Santa Monica, California: Rand Graduate Institute, 1974.

23   Valman B. Cited by Morris N. Editorial boards. *Earth and Life Science Editing* 1985; 24:15.

24   Anonymous. Are referees a good thing? [Editorial]. *Can Med Assoc J* 1974;111:897–8.

25   Douglas-Wilson I. Editorial review: peerless pronouncements. *N Engl J Med* 1977;296:877.

26   Roe IL. Peer review. *American Journal of Medical Technology* 1978;44:365.

27   Belshaw C. Peer review and the *Current Anthropology* experience. *Behavioral and Brain Sciences* 1982;5:200–1.

28   Smigell EO, Ross HL. Factors in the editorial decision. *American Sociologist* 1970;5:19–21.

29   Moossy J, Moossy YR. Anonymous authors, anonymous referees: an editorial exploration. *Journal of Neuropathology and Experimental Neurology* 1985;44:225–8.

30   Knox FG. No unanimity about anonymity. *J Lab Clin Med* 1981;97:1–3.

31   Glen JW, Königsson L-K. Refereeing in earth science journals. *Earth and Life Science Editing* 1976;3:11–13.

32   Waksman BLKH. Information overload in immunology: possibly solutions to the problem of excessive publication. *J Immunol* 1980;124:1009–15.

33   Ziman J. Journal guidelines. *Nature* 1975;258:284.

34   Anonymous. Do scientific journals need a code of practice? [Editorial]. *Nature* 1975;258:1.

35   Patterson K. Bailar JC,III. A review of journal peer review. In: Warren KS, ed. *Selectivity in information systems: survival of the fittest.* New York:Praeger, 1985;64–82.

36   Gordon M. *A study of the evaluation of research papers by primary journals in the UK.* Leicester: Primary Communications Research Centre, 1978.

37   European Life Science Editors' Association. On refereeing in scientific periodicals, 1970. Cited by Glen and Königsson (31)

38   Relman AS, Rennie D, Angell M. Greetings—with regrets. *N Engl J Med* 1980;303:1527–8.

References

39   Wilson JD. Peer review and publication. *J Clin Invest* 1978;58:1697–1701.

40   Bonjean CM, Hullum J. Reasons for journal rejection: an analysis of 600 manuscripts. *PS* 1978;480–3.

41   Anonymous. The refereeing system in the *Journal of Endocrinology* [Editorial]. *J Endocr* 1978;76:9–10.

42   Fulginiti VA. On the editorial process in the medical literature. *Am J Dis Childh* 1984;138:337–9.

43   Yankauer A. Editor's report: peer review. *American Journal of Public Health* 1979;69:222–3.

44   Parker G, Barnett B, Holmes S, Manicavasagar v. Publishing in the parish. *Australian and New Zealand Journal of Psychiatry* 1984;18:78–85.

45   Dehmer P. APS refereeing procedures. *Physics Today* 1982;35:996–7.

46   Ziman J. *Public knowledge.* Cambridge: Cambridge University Press, 1968.

47   Relman AS. Are journals really quality filters? In: Goffman W, Bruer JT, Warren KS, eds. *Research on selective information systems.* New York: Rockefeller Foundation, 1980.

48   Peters DP, Ceci SJ. Peer review practices of psychological journals: the fate of published articles, submitted again. *Behavioral and Brain Sciences* 1982;5:187–95.

49   Harnad S. Peer commentary on peer review. *Behavioural and Brain Sciences* 1982;5:185–6.

50   Peters DP, Ceci SJ. A manuscript masquerade. How well does the review process work? *Sciences* 1980;20:16–9.

51   Cherfas J. Only the names have been changed to protect . . . whom? *New Scientist* 1980;20 March:950.

52   Colman AM. Manuscript evaluation by journal referees and editors: randomness or bias? *Behavioural and Brain Sciences* 1982;5:205–6.

53   Merton R. *The sociology of science.* Chicago: University of Chicago Press, 1973.

54   Zuckerman H. *Scientific elite: Nobel laureates in the United States.* New York: Free Press, 1977.

55   Rosenthal R. Reliability and bias in peer-review practices. *Behavioral and Brain Sciences* 1982;5:235–6.

56   Mahoney MJ. Publication prejudices: an experimental study of confirmatory bias in the peer review system. *Cognitive Therapy and Research* 1977;1:161–75.

57   Perlman D. Reviewer "bias": do Peters and Ceci protest too much? *Behavioral and Brain Sciences* 1982;5:231–2.

58   Relman AS. Dealing with conflicts of interest. *N Engl J Med* 1984;311:405.

References

59   Altman LK. Dealing with conflicts of interest. *N Engl J Med* 1984;311:405.

60   Cohen SN. Dealing with conflicts of interest. *N Engl J Med* 1984;311:404.

61   Goldstone RA. Dealing with conflicts of interest. *N Engl J Med* 1984;311:404.

62   Nightingale SD, Ansell D, Cohen M, *et al.* Dealing with conflicts of interest. *N Engl J Med* 1984;311:405.

63   Relman AS. Dealing with conflicts of interest. *N Engl J Med* 1984;310:1182–3.

64   Maddox J. Privacy and the peer-review system. *Nature* 1984; 312:497.

65   Fleiss JL. Deception in the study of the peer-review process. *Behavioural and Brain Sciences* 1982;5:210–1.

66   Millman, J. Making the plausible implausible: a favorable review of Peters and Ceci's target article. *Behavioural and Brain Sciences* 1982;5:225–6.

67   Mindick B. When we practice to deceive: the ethics of a metascientific inquiry. *Behavioural and Brain Sciences* 1982; 5:226–7.

68   DeBakey L. Authorship and manuscript reviewing: the risk of bias. *Behavioural and Brain Sciences* 1982;5:208–9.

69   Beyer JM. Explaining an unsurprising demonstration: high rejection rates and scarcity of space. *Behavioural and Brain Sciences* 1982;5:202–3.

70   Presser S. Reviewer reliability: confusing random error with systematic error or bias. *Behavioural and Brain Sciences* 1982; 5:223–4.

71   Lazarus D. Interreferee agreement and acceptance rates in physics. *Behavioural and Brain Sciences* 1982;5:219.

72   Glenn ND. The journal article review process as a game of chance. *Behavioural and Brain Sciences* 1982;5:211–2.

73   Geen RG. Review bias: positive or negative, good or bad? *Behavioural and Brain Sciences* 1982;5:211.

74   Whitehurst GJ. The quandary of manuscript reviewing. *Behavioural and Brain Sciences* 1982;5:241–2.

75   Witt JC, Hannafin MJ. Experimenter and reviewer bias. *Behavioural and Brain Sciences* 1982;5:243–4.

76   Majerus P. Journals as filters or sponges. *N Engl J Med* 1978;299:1139.

77   Yankauer A. Peering at peer review. *CBE Views* 1985;8:7–10.

78   Mundy DJ. Time needed for publication of journal articles. *Ann Intern Med* 1984;100:61–2.

79   Dudley HAF. Surgical research: master or servant? *Am J Surg* 1978;135:458–60.

References

80   Goldman L, Loscalzo A. Fate of cardiology research originally published in abstract form. *N Engl J Med* 1980;303:255–9.

81   Strang LB. Abstracts—are they really a dud currency? *Arch Dis Childh* 1984;59:902.

82   International Committee of Medical Journal Editors. Multiple publication. *Br Med J* 1984;288:52.

83   Anonymous. Abstracts—false science. [Editorial]. *Arch Dis Childh* 1984;59:497.

84   Garfield E. *Citation indexing: its theory and application in science, technology, and humanities.* New York: John Wiley, 1979.

85   Garfield E. The Institute for Scientific Information. In: Warren KS, ed. *Coping with the biomedical literature.* New York: Praeger, 1981,183–98.

86   Lock SP. Information overload: solution by quality? *Br Med J* 1982;284:1289–90.

87   Small HG. *Characteristics of frequently cited papers in chemistry.* Philadelphia: ISI, 1974.

88   Lock SP. Repetitive publication: a waste that must stop. *Br Med J* 1984;288:661–2.

89   Abelson P. Excessive zeal to publish. *Science* 1982;218:953.

90   Rubin DB. Rejection, rebuttal, revision: some flexible features of peer review. *Behavioural and Brain Sciences* 1982;5:236–7.

91   Hogan R. The insufficiencies of methodological inadequacy. *Behavioural and Brain Sciences* 1982;5:216.

92   Ziman J. Bias, incompetence, or bad management? *Behavioural and Brain Sciences* 1982;5:245–6.

93   Eckberg DL. Theoretical implications of failure to detect prepublished submissions. *Behavioural and Brain Sciences* 1982;5:209–10.

94   Wilson MA. Research on peer-review practices: problems of interpretation, application, and propriety. *Behavioural and Brain Sciences* 1982;5:242–3.

95   Beaver D deB. On the failure to detect previously published research. *Behavioural and Brain Sciences* 1982;5:199–200.

96   Benichoux R. English as an international language. *Earth and Life Science Editing* 1985;24:8.

97   Thomas GJ. Perhaps it was right to reject the resubmitted manuscripts. *Behavioural and Brain Sciences* 1982;5:240.

98   Anonymous. Must plagiarism thrive? *Br Med J* 1980;281:41–2.

99   Wheelock EF. Plagiarism and freedom of information laws. *Lancet* 1980;i:826.

100 Broad W, Wade N. *Betrayers of the truth.* New York: Simon and Schuster, 1983;94–5.

101 Schor S, Karten I. Statistical evaluation of medical journal manuscripts. *JAMA* 1966;195:1123–8.

102 Gore SM, Jones IG, Rytter EC. Misuse of statistical methods: critical assessment of articles in *BMJ* from January to March 1976. *Br Med J* 1977;i:85–7.

103 Altman D. Improving the quality of statistics in medical journals. In: Gore SM, Altman D. *Statistics in practice.* London: British Medical Association, 1982;21–4.

104 DerSimonian R, Charette J, McPeek B, Mosteller F. Reporting on methods in clinical trials. *N Engl J Med* 1982;306:1332–6.

105 Lionel NDW, Herxheimer A. Assessing reports of therapeutic trials. *Br Med J* 1970;iii:637–40.

106 Venulet J, Blattern R, von Bulow J, Berneker GC. How good are articles on adverse drug reactions? *Br Med J* 1982;284:252–4.

107 Altman L, Melcher L. Fraud in science. *Br Med J* 1983;286:2003–6.

108 Broad WJ. Imbroglio at Yale. I. Emergence of a fraud. II. A top job lost. *Science* 1980;210:38–41,171–3.

109 Budiansky S. False date confessed. *Nature* 1983;301:101.

110 Budiansky S. Food and drug data fudged. *Nature* 1983;302:560.

111 Budiansky S. NIH withdraws research grant. *Nature* 1983;309:738.

112 Anonymous. In Bristol now. *Nature* 1983;294:509.

113 Angell M. Editors and fraud. *CBE Views* 1983;6:3–8.

114 Majerus P. Fraud in medical research. *J Clin Invest* 1982;70:213–7.

115 Horrobin DF. Peer review: a philosophically faulty concept which is proving disastrous for science. *Behavioural and Brain Sciences* 1982;5:217–8.

116 Ingelfinger FJ. Charity and peer review in publication. *N Engl J Med* 1975;293:1371–2.

117 Pickard WF. Role of the referee. *Physics Today* 1982;35:114.

118 Cohen J. A coefficient of agreement for nominal scales. *Educational and Psychological Measurement* 1960;20:37–46.

119 Tuchman B. *Practising history.* London: Macmillan, 1982.

120 Martin BR, Irvine J. CERN: past performance and future prospects. 1. CERN's position in world high-energy physics. *Research Policy* 1984;13:183–210.

121 Bailar JC, Patterson K. Journal peer review: the need for a research agenda. *N Engl J Med* 1985;312:65407.

122 Garfield E. To remember Sir Hans Krebs: novelist, friend, and adviser. *Current Contents* 1982;31:5–11.

123 Powell E. *Medicine and politics: 1975 and after.* London:Pitman Medical, 1976.

124 Kellenberger E. Alternatives to peer review. *Trends Biochem Sci* 1981;6:11.

125 Abelson P. Information exchange groups. *Science* 1966;154:727.

References

126 Doermann AH, Gallant JA, McCarthy BJ, Morris DR, Nester E, Rutter WJ, *et al.* IEG's: some evaluations. *Science* 1966;154:332–6.

127 Dray S. Information exchange group No 5. *Science* 1966; 153:694–5.

128 Confrey EA. Information exchange groups to be discontinued. *Science* 1966;154:843.

129 Boffey PM. Psychology: apprehension over a new communications system. *Science* 1970;167:1228–30.

130 Anonymous. Plagiarism, piracy and principles [Editorial]. *Nature* 1980;286:831–2.

131 Dickson D. Harvard guidelines for avoiding fraud. *Nature* 1982;295:271.

132 Association of American Medical Colleges. *The maintenance of high ethical standards in the conduct of research. Report of an ad hoc committee adopted by the executive council of the AAMC 24 June 1982.* Washington, DC: AAMC, 1982.

133 Norman C. No fraud found in alcoholism study. *Science* 1982;218:771.

134 Kuhn T. *The structure of scientific revolutions.* 2nd edn. Chicago: University of Chicago Press, 1970.

135 Relman AS. How reliable are letters? *N Engl J Med* 1983;308:1219–20.

136 Yates FE. Scientific creativity, pathological science, and the gauntlet of review. *American Journal of Physiology* 1979;5:R1–3.

137 Barber B. Resistance by scientists to scientific discovery. *Science* 1961;134:596–602.

138 Yalow RS. Radioimmunoassay: a probe for the fine structure of biologic systems. *Science* 1978;200:1236–45.

139 Yalow RS. Competency testing for reviewers and editors. *Behavioural and Brain Sciences* 1982;5:244–5.

140 Ruderfer M. The fallacy of peer review—judgment without science and a case history. *Speculations in Science and Technology* 1980;3:533–62.

141 Angell M. Fraud in science. *Science* 1983;219:1417–8.

142 Price D de S. Script of talk for IFSEA meeting, Rehovot, Israel, 1982. Philadelphia:IFSEA.

143 Marinov S. *The thorny way of truth.* Graz, Austria:Est-Ovest, 1982.

144 Anonymous. Unorthodox assessments [Editorial]. *Nature* 1982;300:566.

145 Evans M. *Janáček's tragic operas.* London: Faber and Faber, 1977.

146 King DW, McDonald DD, Roder NK. *Scientific journals in the United States: their production, use, and economics.* Stroudsburg, Pa: Hutchinson Ross, 1981. Cited by Bailar and Patterson (121).

147   Michel FC. Solving the problem of refereeing. *Physics Today* 1982;35:9,82.

148   Anonymous. Monument for a giant. *Nature* 1981;294:296.

149   Krebs H. *Reminiscences and reflections.* Oxford: Clarendon Press, 1981.

150   Medawar PB. Anglo-Saxon attitudes. *Encounter* 1965;25:52–8.

151   Taegtmeyer H. Scientific journals: evaluation of evolution. *N Engl J Med* 1981;305:1353–4.

152   Hutchison R. Medical literature. *Lancet* 1939;ii:1059–62.

153   Durack DT. The weight of medical knowledge. *N Engl J Med* 1978;298:773–5.

154   Strub RL, Black FW. Multiple authorship. *Lancet* 1976,ii:1090–1.

155   Price D de S. Ethics of scientific publication. *Science* 1964;144:665–7.

156   Ziman J. The proliferation of scientific literature: a natural process. *Science* 1980;208:369–71.

157   Branscomb LM. Misinformation explosion: is the literature worth reviewing? *Scientific Research* 1968;3:49–56.

158   Goffman W. The ecology of the biomedical literature and information retrieval. In: Warren KS, ed. *Coping with the biomedical literature.* New York: Praeger, 1981;31–46.

159   Rossner S. Key words: publication practice. *Eur J Clin Pharmacol* 1984;26:283.

160   Warren KS, Goffman W. The ecology of the medical literatures. *Am J Med Sci* 1972;263:267–73.

161   Huth EJ. An information system for the future? *Ann Intern Med* 1980;93:139–40.

162   Bernstein LM, Siegel ER, Goldstein CM. The hepatitis knowledge base: a prototype information transfer system. *Ann Intern Med* 1980;93:169–81.

163   Scientific Information Committee of the Royal Society. *A study of the scientific information system in the United Kingdom.* London: The Royal Society, 1981.

164   Berry EM. The evolution of scientific and medical journals. *N Engl J Med* 1981;305:400–2.

165   Glenn J. The academic surgeon: a young surgeon's perspective. *Surgery* 1984;12:123–4.

166   Irwin St, Roy AD. Published or be damned! *Lancet* 1984;ii:859.

167   Safran C. The weight of medical knowledge. *N Engl J Med* 1978;299:263.

168   Warren KS. The weight of medical knowledge. *N Engl J Med* 1978;299:263.

169   Windsor D. The weight of medical knowledge. *N Engl J Med* 1978;299:263.

References

170   Berger SA. The weight of medical knowledge. *N Engl J Med* 1978;299:263.

171   Dan B. The paper chase. *JAMA* 1983;249:2872–3.

172   Smith RJ. Scientific fraud probed at AAAS meeting. *Science* 1985;228:1292–3.

173   Knox S. Deeper problems for Darsee: Emory probe. *JAMA* 1983;249:2867–76.

174   Crosland S. *Tony Crosland.* London: Cape, 1982.

175   Stossel TP. Speed: an essay on biomedical communication. *N Engl J Med* 1985;312:123–6.

176   Douglas-Wilson I. *Twilight of the medical journal?* BMA annual scientific meeting, Hull, 1974. London: BMA.

177   Gustafson T. Why doesn't Soviet science do better than it does? In: Lubrano L, Solomon SG, eds. *The social context of Soviet science.* Boulder, Colorado: Westview Press, 1980;31–68.

178   Commoner B. Peering at peer review. *Hospital Practice* 1978; November:25,29.

179   Curzon G. The need for fairer methods of assessment. *Times Higher Educational Supplement* 1982;22 October:14.

180   Irvine J. Martin BR. What direction for basic scientific research? In: Gibbons M, Gummett P, Udgaonkar BM, eds. *Science and technology policy in the 1980s and beyond.* London: Longman, 1984;67–98.

181   Medical Research Council. *Annual report. 1983–84.* London: MRC, 1984.

182   Irvine J, Martin BR. CERN: past performance and future prospects.2. The scientific performance of the CERN accelerators. *Research Policy* 1984;13:247–84.

183   Osmond DH. Malice's wonderland: research funding and peer review. *Journal of Neurobiology* 1983;14:95–112.

184   Nelson K. Reliability, bias or quality: what is the issue? *Behavioral and Brain Sciences* 1982;5:219–20.

185   Louttit RT. Peer review: prediction of the future or judgement of the past? *Behavioral and Brain Sciences* 1982;5:219–20.

186   'ES'. The confidentiality and anonymity of assessment. *Minerva* 1975;13:341–8.

187   Clark AH. Luck, merit, and peer review. *Science* 1982;215:11.

188   Horrobin DF. Personal view. *Br Med J* 1974;iv:463.

189   Irvine J, Martin B, Oldham G. *Research evaluation in British science: a SPURU review.* Brighton: Science Policy Research Unit, 1983.

190   Committee on Biomedical Research in the Veterans Administration. In: *Biomedical research in the Veterans Administration.* Washington, DC: National Academy of Sciences, 1977.

191   Horrobin DF. The business of research. *Lancet* 1972;i:273.

References

192   Horrobin DF. Referees and research administrators: barriers to scientific research? *Br Med J* 1974;ii:216–8.

193   Michie D. Peer review and the bureaucracy. *Times Higher Education Supplement* 1978;4 August:12.

194   Horrobin D. In praise of non-experts. *New Scientist* 1982;24 June:843–4.

195   Gustafson T. The controversy over peer review. *Science* 1975;190:1060–5.

196   Apirion D. Research funding and the peer review system. *Fed Proc* 1979;38:2649–50.

197   Roy R. Alternative to peer review? *Science* 1981;212:1377.

198   Jacobs LS. Alternative to peer review? *Science* 1981;212:1337.

199   Kalt MR. Alternative to peer review. *Science* 1981;212:1337.

200   McCreery RL. Alternative to peer review? *Science* 1981;212:1336.

201   Easter SS. Alternative to peer review? *Science* 1981;212:1337.

202   Morawetz H. Alternative to peer review? *Science* 1981;212:1337.

203   Birnbaum H. Alternative to peer review? *Science* 1981;212:1337.

204   Berns MW. Alternative to peer review? *Science* 1981;212;1337–8.

205   Roy R. Alternative to peer review? *Science* 1981;212:1338–9.

206   Noble JH. Peer review: quality control or applied social research. *Science* 1974;185:916–21.

207   Cole S, Cole JR, Simon GA. Chance and consensus in peer review. *Science* 1981;214:1886.

208   Cole JR, Cole S. Which researcher will get the grant? *Nature* 1979;279:575–6.

209   Martin BR, Irvine J. CERN: past performance and future prospects. 3. CERN and the future of world high-energy physics. *Research Policy* 1984;13:311–42.

210   Nelkin D. Intellectual property: the control of scientific information. *Science* 1982;216:704–8.

211   Melnick JL. Journal guidelines. *Nature* 1975;259:264.

212   Bradford Hill A. The reasons for writing. *Br Med J* 1965;ii:870–1.

213   Brain WR. Structure of the scientific paper. *Br Med J* 1965;ii:868–9.

214   Lock SP. *Thorne's better medical writing.* 2nd ed. Tunbridge Wells: Pitman Medical, 1977.

215   O'Connor M, Woodford P. *Writing scientific papers in English.* Amsterdam: Associated Scientific Publishers, 1975.

216   Hawkins CF. *Speaking and writing in medicine.* Springfield, Illinois: Charles C Thomas, 1967.

217   Huth EJ. *How to write and publish papers in the medical sciences.* Philadelphia: ISI, 1982.

References

218 Smith R. Steaming up windows and refereeing medical papers. *Br Med J* 1982;285:1259–61.

219 Bishop CT. The review process. In: *How to edit a scientific journal.* Philadelphia: ISI, 1984.

220 O'Connor M. *Editing scientific books and journals.* Tunbridge Wells: Pitman Medical, 1978.

221 Sommers HS. Improving refereeing. *Physics Today* 1973; 36:92–3.

222 Relman AS. The Ingelfinger rule. *N Engl J Med* 1981; 305:824–6.

223 Donaldson RM. Exclusive publication. *Gastroenterology* 1976; 70:811–2.

224 International Committee of Medical Journal Editors. Guidelines on authorship. *Br Med J* 1985;291:722.

225 Anonymous. Abuses of authorship [Editorial]. *Ann Intern Med* 1984;100:147–8.

226 Burman K. Hanging from the masthead: reflections on authorship. *Ann Intern Med* 1982;97:602–5.

227 Anonymous. Responsibilities of coauthorship [Editorial]. *Ann Intern Med* 1983;99:266–7.

228 World Medical Association. Human experimentation: code of ethics of the World Medical Association. Declaration of Helsinki. *Br Med J* 1964;ii:177.

229 Altman DG. Statistics in medical journals. *Statistics in Medicine* 1982;i:59–71.

230 Altman DG, Gore SM, Gardner MJ, Pocock SJ. Statistical guidelines for contributors to medical journals. *Br Med J* 1983;286:1489–93.

231 Schor S. Statistical reviewing program for medical manuscripts. *American Statistician* 1967;21:28–31.

232 Gardner MJ, Altman DG, Jones DR, Machin D. Is the statistical assessment of papers submitted to the *British Medical Journal* effective? *Br Med J* 1983;286:1485–8.

233 Gardner MJ, Machin D, Campbell MJ. Use of checklists for the assessment of the statistical content of medical studies. *Br Med J* 1985 (in press).

234 Mosteller F. Evaluation: requirements for scientific proof. In: Warren KS, ed. *Coping with the biomedical literature.* New York: Praeger, 1981;103–21.

235 DerSimonian R, Charette J, McPeek B, Mosteller F. Reporting on methods in clinical trials. *N Engl J Med* 1983;308:597.

236 Sackett DL. Evaluation: requirements for clinical application. In: Warren KS, ed. *Coping with the biomedical literature.* New York: Praeger, 1981;123–57.

237 Simon R, Wittes RE. Methodologic guidelines for reports of clinical trials. *Cancer Treatment Reports* 1985;69:1–3.

References

238   Anonymous. Criteria for journal reports of suspected adverse drug reactions [Editorial]. *Clinical Pharmacol* 1982;i:554–5.

239   Berneker GC, Ciucci AG, Joyce J. Standards for reporting adverse drug reactions. *Br Med J* 1983;287:1720.

240   Anonymous. Improving reports of adverse drug reactions. *Br Med J* 1984;289:898.

241   Fowler J, O'Connor M. Refereeing, commissioning and editing for journals and books. *Earth and Life Science Editing* 1980;11:10–12.

242   Cicchetti DV. On peer review: "We have met the enemy and he is us." *Behavioural and Brain Science* 1982;5:205.

243   Böttiger LE. Reference lists in medical journals—language and length. *Acta Medica Scand* 1983;214:73–7.

244   Böttiger LE. Reflections on references. *Acta Med Scand* 1983;214:1–2.

245   Harnad S. Peer commentary on peer review: a case study in scientific quality control. *Behavioural and Brain Sciences* 1982;5:185–6.

246   Gordon MD. Maintaining quality: refereeing. *Earth and Life Science Editing* 1978;6:12–13.

247   Honig WM. Peer review in the physical sciences: an editor's view. *Behavioural and Brain Sciences* 1982;5:216–7.

248   Crandall R. Editorial responsibilities in manuscript review. *Behavioural and Brain Sciences* 1982;5:207–8.

249   Scarr S. Anosmic peer review: a rose by another name is evidently not a rose. *Behavioural and Brain Sciences* 1982;5:237–8.

250   Morgan PP. Anonymity in medical journals. *Can Med Assoc J* 1984;121:1007–8.

251   Palermo DS. Biases, decisions and auctorial rebuttal in the peer-review process. *Behavioural and Brain Sciences* 1982;5:230–1.

252   Armstrong JS. Barriers to scientific contributions: the author's formula. *Behavioural and Brain Sciences* 1982;5:197–9.

253   Chubin DE. Peer review and the courts: notes of a participant-scientist. *Bull Sci Tech Soc* 1982;2:423–32.

254   Robertson P. Towards open refereeing. *New Scientist* 1976;71:410.

255   Ziman J. Journal guidelines. Nature 1976;259:264.

256   Soffer A. Identification of reviewers: a statement of policy. *Chest* 1979;75:295–6.

257   Woolf P. Fraud in science: how much, how serious? *Hastings Center Report* 1981;11:9–14.

258   Goodstein LD. When will the editors start to edit? *Behavioural and Brain Sciences* 1982;5:212–3.

259   Gordon M. *Running a refereeing system.* Leicester: University of Leicester Primary Communications Research Centre, 1983.

References

260 Stossel TP. Reviewer status and review quality: experience of the *Journal of Clinical Investigation*. *N Engl J Med* 1985;312:658–9.

261 Soffer A. The unique role of peer review journals. *Chest* 1980;78:547–8.

262 Tax S, Rubinstein RA. Responsibility in reviewing and research. *Behavioural and Brain Sciences* 1982;5:238–40.

263 Cameron E, Pauling L. Supplemental ascorbate in the supportive treatment of cancer. *Proc Natl Acad Sci USA* 1976; 73:3685–9;1978;75:4538–42. (Comment. Comroe JH, Jr. *Proc Natl Acad Sci USA* 1978;75:4543.)

264 Relman AS. Editorial review. *N Engl J Med* 1982;307;899.

265 Bernard HR. Computer-assisted referee selection as a means of reducing potential editorial bias. *Behavioural and Brain Sciences* 1982;5:202.

266 Scientific Information Committee of the Royal Society. *Quality and economics of scientific journals.* London: The Royal Society, 1975.

267 Lock SP. Brave new journals: 2033. *Finnish Medical Journal* 1983;38:935–8.

268 Elia JJ, jr. Another medium for the *Journal. N Engl J Med* 1984;311:1631.

269 Lock SP. Two cheers for the computer? *Br Med J* 1985; 290:1609–10.

270 Anonymous. Computers that speed the news of science. *Business Week* 1982;25 January:36F.

271 Gastel B. The review process. *CBE Views* 1984;7:18–21.

272 *Clinical Notes On-Line.* Lancaster: Elsevier-IRCS, 1985.

273 Anonymous. Unconventional publication [Editorial]. *Br Med J* 1973;i:631.

274 Horrobin DF. Unconventional publication. *Br Med J* 1973; i:801–2.

275 Garfield E. More on scientific journals. *N Engl J Med* 1982; 307:506.

276 Crean J. *Famous last words.* London: Omnibus, 1979.

277 Saxov S. Is the referee the editor's evil genius? *Earth and Life Science Editing* 1981;12:7–8.

278 *Oxford English Dictionary. Compact edition.* Oxford: Oxford University Press, 1971.

279 Burchfield RE, ed. Peer. *Supplement to the Oxford English Dictionary. Vol iii O-Scz.* Oxford: Oxford University Press, 1981;343.

280 Mencken HL. *The American language.* New York: Knopf, 1977.

281 Vercueil AE. Peer review. *S Afr Med J* 1984;65:863–4.

INDEX

Index

Betrayers of the Truth. 49, 53
Betterment: definition. 108
Bias. *See under* Referees
Big Science. 104, 105
Blemish: definition. 23
Boyle, Robert. 'Philosophicall robbery'. 21, 54
Bradford Hill, Sir Austin. vii
British Medical Journal
  Acceptance rate. 59
  Hanging committee. 8
  Impact factor. 58
  Page cost. 129
  Statistical errors study. 50
  Statistics checklist. 115 (table)
  for clinical trials. 116 (table)
  Survey. 56
    acceptance and authors' qualifications. 61 (table)
    acceptance rate. 59
    accepted papers citations. 58
    consensus. 64, 68
    difficulties. 70
    gold standard. 66
    proportion of papers rejected/accepted. 64 (table)
    recommendations. 68
    referee bias. 61
    referee status. 62 (table)
    rejected articles outcome. 61, 63 (table), 64 (table)
    results/comments. 59
    statistical evaluation. 59
    submitted papers, fate. 60 (table)
  'Unreviewed Reports'. 75
Burt, Sir Cyril. 51

Causation. Cancer trials: checklist. 118 (table)
CERN
  Annual budget. 93
  Assessment. 105
Charlemagne. 142 (Appendix II)
Checklists. 116, 117, 118 (tables)
  Value. 120, 131
China. Peer review in. 3
Citations
  Analysis. 13

  history. 13
  research grant applications. 101
  value. 13
Articles accepted/rejected by *BMJ*. 64 (table)
Fundamental references. 12
Number, annual. 13
Patterns. Chapter 4, note 1
Quickest abstracts. 12
Rates: institutional prestige and. 29
Referees' comments, correlations. 43
Time lapse. 12
Weighting factors. Chapter 8, note 3
Clegg, Hugh. vi
Clinical Notes On-Line. 136 (Appendix I)
Clinical trials
  Acceptability. 51
  Cancer causation: checklist. 118 (table)
  Randomised double-blind controlled. 79
  Statistics. 50
  BMJ checklist. 116 (table)
Computers
  Data bases: updating information. Chapter 6, note 9
  Electronic journals. 135 (Appendix I)
  Information retrieval. 135 (Appendix I)
  Referees, choosing by. 130
Comtec Corporation. 135 (Appendix I)
Confidentiality over peer review. Chapter 7, note 3
Consensus
  BMJ survey. 64, 65 (table)
  Filtration by. Chapter 6, note 9
  Over-emphasis. 69
'Converging partial indicators'. 105
Copyright. 45
Correlation: definition. 93
Correspondence
  Alternatives to peer review for research funds. 98
  Evaluation by. 43
  Statistical error detection and. 50
  Unreviewed. 75
Cort, Joseph. 53
Council of Biology Editors. 135 (Appendix I)

Index

Index

Index

Index

Index